Creative Social Work in Health Care

Helen Rehr, DSW, Professor of Community Medicine Emerita and consultant on social-health research, education, and program planning to the Department of Social Work Services and the Division of Social Work, The Mount Sinai School of Medicine and Medical Center. Dr. Rehr received a bachelor's degree from Hunter College and a master's degree and doctorate from the Columbia University School of Social Work. She is the recipient of an honorary degree of Doctor of Science from Hunter College. She has been Edith J. Baerwald Professor of Community Medicine (Social Work), Mount Sinai School of Medicine and Adjunct Clinical Professor, Hunter College School of Social Work and the Brookdale Center on Aging, Hunter College. Dr. Rehr was Director of the Department of Social Work Services, the Division of Social Work (Community Medicine), and the Brookdale Center for Continuous Education, The Mount Sinai School of Medicine, CUNY. She is a Fellow of the Gerontological Society of America, a Fellow of the Brookdale Center on Aging, and a Fellow of the New York Academy of Medicine. Dr. Rehr has been awarded numerous honors, including election to the Hunter College Hall of Fame; Distinguished Social Work Practitioner of the National Academies of Practice; the Knee-Wittman Award for Lifetime Achievement; and the Ida M. Cannon Award of the Society of Hospital Social Work Directors, the American Hospital Association. Dr. Rehr is the author, coauthor, and editor of more than 100 published studies, reports, monographs, articles, chapters, and books. She has been a trustee of the New York Foundation and a member of the Board of Directors of the Scholarship and Welfare Fund of Hunter College. She is a member of the Board of the Center for the Study of Social Work Practice, Columbia University School of Social Work. She has held visiting professorships in Israel and Australia, and was the Kenneth L. Pray Visiting Professor at the University of Pennsylvania School of Social Work.

Gary Rosenberg, PhD, is the Edith J. Baerwald Professor of Community Medicine (Social Work) and Senior Vice President, The Mount Sinai Medical Center, where he also was Director of the Department of Social Work Services. Dr. Rosenberg received a bachelor's degree from Hunter College, a master's in social work from Adelphi University, and his doctorate from New York University. Dr. Rosenberg has been awarded numerous honors, including election to the Hunter College Hall of Fame and named Distinguished Social Work Practitioner of the National Academies of Practice and Outstanding Alumni, Adelphi University. He also received the Founder's Day Award, New York University. He is a Fellow of the Brookdale Center on Aging and a Fellow of the New York Academy of Medicine. He is a recipient of the Ida M. Cannon Award of the Society for Hospital Social Work Directors, the American Hospital Association, and a past president of the Society. Dr. Rosenberg is editor in chief of the peer-reviewed journal, *Social Work in Health Care*. He has written a number of books and numerous articles.

Susan Blumenfield, DSW, is Director, Department of Social Work Services, The Mount Sinai Medical Center; Associate Director, Mount Sinai Hospital; and Associate Professor, The Mount Sinai School of Medicine. Dr. Blumenfield received a bachelor's degree, with distinction, from Cornell University, a master's in social work from Columbia University School of Social Work, and her doctorate from the Hunter College School of Social Work. Dr. Blumenfield is a recipient of the UJA Federation Rose Zeitlin Goldstein Award and has been elected to the Hunter College Hall of Fame. She is a Fellow of the Brookdale Center on Aging and a Diplomate of the American Board of Examiners in Clinical Social Work. Dr. Blumenfield has been awarded a number of grants for practice and research studies, is the author of numerous journal articles and book chapters, and has been invited frequently to speak at national and international conferences and seminars. She is a member of the editorial board of the *Journal of Gerontological Social Work*.

Creative Social Work in Health Care
Clients, The Community, and Your Organization

Helen Rehr, DSW
Gary Rosenberg, PhD
Susan Blumenfield, DSW
Editors

Springer Publishing Company

Springer Publishing Company, Inc.
536 Broadway
New York, NY 10012-3955

Cover design by Janet Joachim
Acquisitions Editor: Bill Tucker
Production Editor: Kathleen Kelly

98 99 00 01 02 / 5 4 3 2 1

Library of Congress Cataloging-in-Publication Data

Rehr, Helen.
    Creative social work in health care : clients, the community, and your organization / Helen Rehr, Gary Rosenberg, Susan Blumenfield.
       p.   cm.
    Includes bibliographical references (p.   ) and index.
    ISBN 0-8261-1199-8
    1. Mount Sinai Hospital (New York, N.Y.) Dept. of Social Work Services—History. 2. Medical social work—New York (State)—New York—History. 3. Medical social work—Research—New York (State)—New York. I. Rosenberg, Gary. II. Blumenfield, Susan.
III. Title.
HV687.5.U5R45   1998
364.1′0425—DC21   97-53579
                                                CIP

Printed in the United States of America

In recognition of the 90th anniversary of the Department of Social Work Services (created in 1906), this book is a tribute to the professional social workers whose publications reflect on their service, education, and research over a period of 40 years.

Contents

Contributors

Claire Bennett, MSW, Consultant, Department of Social Work Services; Lecturer, Department of Community Medicine (Social Work); Mount Sinai Medical Center, New York, NY.

Barbara Brenner, DrPh, Director, Department of Community Relations; Instructor, Department of Community Medicine (Social Work); Mount Sinai Medical Center, New York, NY.

Myrna I. Lewis, MSW, Assistant Professor, Department of Community Medicine (Social Work); Mount Sinai Medical Center, New York, NY.

Kenneth Peake, MSW, Assistant Director, Adolescent Health Center, Mount Sinai Medical Center, New York, NY.

Nancy Showers, DSW, former Assistant Director, Department of Social Work Services; former Assistant Professor, Department of Community Medicine (Social Work); Mount Sinai Medical Center, New York, NY.

Mary Ellen Siegel, MSW, Lecturer, Department of Community Medicine (Social Work); Mount Sinai Medical Center, New York, NY.

Virginia Walther, MSW, Senior Assistant Director, Department of Social Work Services; Instructor, Department of Community Medicine (Social Work); Mount Sinai Medical Center, New York, NY.

Alma T. Young, EdD, Director of Continuing Education and Quality Assurance (Social Work); Assistant Professor, Department of Community Medicine (Social Work); Mount Sinai Medical Center, New York, NY.

Foreword

The volume with which you are about to become acquainted is timely and unique. It addresses some of the most urgent and daunting challenges that confront social work practice and education; namely, how best to rethink or restructure fundamental aspects of social work and health care in a turbulent, rapidly changing and highly uncertain environment. The authors address these issues skillfully and from a historical perspective that is rooted in a strong and coherent body of scholarship. The prescriptions that they set forth apply directly to social work practice in health care settings. Yet most apply as well to other important venues in which social work is practiced.

Creative Social Work in Health Care is singular also because it is the only publication of its kind in which all of the central findings and recommendations derive not from academia but, rather, from the cumulative work of scores of social work clinicians and administrators. The research-based insights concerning social work practice that appear in this book are grounded in the workaday world of health care service delivery. Whether regarded as the best possible laboratory for knowledge development, or perhaps less glamorously, as the real-world battleground from which practical insights necessarily must spring, this volume demonstrates that research has to be informed by practice, grounded in it, and as often as possible conducted by practitioners in order to optimally improve the services of helping professionals. Such a realization may be sobering for some academics. Yet, it is a lesson that needs to be learned with alacrity.

This book differs from others, too, because of its unique authorship. It is difficult to imagine any trio of authors, based on their extensive experience and expertise, who could better blend sound social work practice—in all of its glorious complexity—with rigorous research so as to advance knowledge development, education, and practice in social work. The authors are intimately acquainted with the individual, community, organization, administrative, and policy aspects of social work practice in health care. Yet, they are equally able and comfortable in the world of social work academia.

Last, but not least, this book is of singular importance because it chronicles the remarkable scholarship and productivity over four decades of the staff at a social work department in a world-class medical setting; namely, the Mount Sinai Medical Center in New York City. This record of scholarship from within a practice setting is perhaps unparalleled in the social work literature. Readers would do well to ponder and, to the extent possible, replicate the factors or circumstances that have yielded such productivity. Whether they inhere in an organizational model, institutional expectations, systemic opportunity structures, individual leadership, or any combination thereof, much can be learned.

It is evident that the longstanding attention accorded to research, evaluation, cost-benefit measurement, and similar issues by this social work department place it substantially ahead of other entities that lag woefully in this regard. The department of social work and the larger medical center are positioned well to adapt to the intellectual, operational, and systemic challenges that confront health care and social work. The achievements of these practitioners and scholars should lead social work educators to ponder anew whether it is prudent to place all or even most of their research and education "eggs" in the single "basket" of social work academia. Certainly the following pages demonstrate that it is possible and, indeed, advisable for social workers to stimulate advances by creating organizational models for research and education that extend beyond the narrow confines of the modern university. In this way, as in many others, the present volume sets forth thought-provoking, well-grounded, and timely considerations that are bound to advance the interrelated worlds of knowledge development, education, and practice in social work and health care.

RONALD A. FELDMAN
Dean and Ottman Centennial Professor
for the Advancement of Social Work Education
Columbia University
New York, New York

Acknowledgments

The editors and contributors gratefully acknowledge the editorial assistance of Maryanne Shanahan and the secretarial help of William Barnes in the preparation of this text.

Acknowledgments

1

Introduction: Practitioners Respond to Clients, Community, and Organization

Helen Rehr, Gary Rosenberg, and Susan Blumenfield

As we prepare to leave the 20th century behind, a vision of health care delivery in the next century is difficult to conjure. What will be the range of social and health care services that are needed, available, and accessible? Who will provide what services? How will providers be paid? Where will the current trend toward managed care and capitation systems lead us? Will everyone have access to care and be able to pay for it? Or will the group of 42 million people without insurance and with limited access to care grow even larger? Where will the profession of social work fit in the schema? Has the profession developed the knowledge, values, and skills that will carry it into the next millennium?

The profession of social work has developed throughout a period of 100 years, its history paralleling that of the profession of medicine, its evolution as a profession with multiple roles and functions occurring most notably in the 50 years since World War II. Advances in science and medicine have been remarkable since then, indeed throughout this century—the incidence of disease reduced, diagnostic and therapeutic directions enhanced, the quality of life improved, and life extended for the severely chronically ill who have limited social, emotional, and financial support systems. Social work practice and the programs the profession developed or to whose development it contributed were influenced greatly by these advances and by the dramatic change in the health care environment since World War II. The shift in the dominance of services from physician to other health care providers as well as competition and deregulation have influenced the nature of health and social services. Limited access to and rationing of services, religious and philosophical beliefs, and individuals' life styles have affected the way social workers now offer services—how, when, where, and to whom. Throughout its history the profession has responded to clients, to the community, and to organizations.

The professional history of social work has not been without turbulence. As it developed and evolved, becoming more adept at multiple roles and functions, developing policy, practice and programs, the profession splintered into many component parts, which dichotomized the clinical area from social policy and practitioners from academics. Although the splintered components might serve particular areas of the profession, they do not integrate the profession. Consequently, social work is not perceived as an entity but as an array of multiple and separate components that function independently; i.e., social work services, social policy, program planning, and social research. Moreover, disparate and controversial directions occur within each component.

Publications in professional social work journals illustrate the wide range of views and the disparity among these views, even within specializations. Because social work academics appear to be the major source of articles, the question arises as to whether a difference exists between the published articles of social work practitioners and those of social work academics.

THE QUESTION

We asked: If a social work department in a health care setting assessed its collected publications, would those publications mirror the environment of the profession (i.e., the splintering and dichotomy), or would integration and logical directions related to societal concerns and social needs be apparent in the department's programs and practices? We speculated whether published writings by department practitioners had 1) responded to clients, the community, and the organization; 2) contributed in a meaningful way to the profession's literature; 3) contributed to social work's history; and/or 4) enhanced social work practice knowledge in the health care field. We further speculated that, at the very least, a review and analysis of the publications would offer a view over time of practitioners' perceptions of the practice and program issues that had occurred in the health setting. A compilation could illustrate practitioners' services, the programs in which they were involved, and their educational and research endeavors. It also could illustrate the external environment; that is, social-health care in society as a whole. Finally, a review and analysis of publications could reflect changes in social and health care delivery within a major medical setting and in social work in health care. Practically, it could help organize and harness a department's published body of work and track the history of the development of the department's philosophy and direction.

THE REVIEW AND ANALYSIS

This review and analysis encompasses the published work of clinicians and administrators in social-health services at Mount Sinai Medical Center, New York, from 1953 through 1991. It illustrates their practice and experiences, and the wide range of individuals served in a 150-year-old health setting with a history of medical and social work education and research, which provides the full scope of medical and psychiatric care and which has been a formal academic medical school for 30 years. The writings reflect a range of experiences by social workers who depict their practice, clients, and ideas as well as their relationship to the institution; to their colleagues, peers, and other health professionals; to the community; and to the field of health care. The writings also reflect a range of service and educational programs in social work and medicine. Authors are concerned with the ethics of their practice, the institution, and other providers. Through a host of applied studies, practitioners assessed their practice and programs to determine the functional benefits and utility of social-health services to their recipients and to recommend change as needed.

Professional journals and books contain an array of practice and program articles that address specific components of social work services, but content is scattered and no written knowledge base of practice exists. A review and analysis of the collected written work of nearly four decades in one institution should reflect the changes in social work in relation to health care over time. A few reviews have addressed publications of specific subjects and areas of practice that have appeared in social work journals or texts, regardless of the origin of authorship (Berkman, 1978 and Bracht, 1978, social work in health; Davidson & Clarke, 1990, health social work; Germain, 1985, clinical social work; Harbert & Ginsberg, 1979, aging). This review covers the range of subject and topic areas that engaged a teaching hospital's social work practice staff during 40 years.

THE PREMISE

Publications about who writes for professional journals highlight the writings of academics and, largely, the extent to which they publish (Green & Bentley, 1994). These publications suggest that academics in schools of social work produce the most meaningful writings. Most social work academics believe that a theoretical and/or scientific basis for practice should exist. They suggest that research should underpin services with a technical knowledge that would validate them in either a paradigm of problem, process, and outcome or a mosaic of tested formulations. However, for many aspects of practice, clinicians function using the "black-box" principle; that is, the container for the mysterious "somethings" for which no immediate explanation exists because information is not readily at hand. As Schon (1983) suggests, practice is based more on "reflection-in-action."

The authors who wrote between 1953 and 1991 were not, in the main, academics in a school of social work, but were and are social work clinicians and managers with field-related social work and medical educational responsibilities. A few engaged in research in partnership with practice staff, and many were/are actively involved in community programs. In looking at their publications, we asked:

- What has concerned the practitioners who publish?
- What issues have they explored?
- What did they learn from their practice and programs?
- What is their prescription for social work in health care for the future?

THE SOURCE

The list of publications was drawn primarily from annual reports of departmental and faculty activities. Where possible, original publications or abstracts related to publications were obtained. An information form was completed for each publication, noting publication data, subject classification, whether the publication was an applied study and/or funded, whether authorship was interdisciplinary, and whether the publication included a literature review. Information about the professions of coauthors was obtained by examining publications, reviewing medical center listings, and querying authors or others knowledgeable about particular coauthors. Publication source (e.g., peer-reviewed article or book) was noted. Works are included in the review only if the dates of publication occurred during times of appointment to the department within the review period. Some publications appeared in more than one venue and/or in more than one version. Although considered only once for purposes of statistical analysis, all versions are included in the Master List of Publications, which is separated by content area and provided in each of the relevant chapters in this book.

THE CONTENT

In reviewing the collection of published works (of which there were 463, representing 693 subjects), it was logical to find that clinical interventions and social work roles and functions would represent more than 25% (173) of the 693 subjects in the compilation. Program development and social-health care delivery followed with 14% (97) of the total subjects; in this area, social work authors describe and assess the programs in which they were clinically involved. Social workers' roles in education (11.3%) were illustrated in three primary areas—articles for social work students (41); articles for practicing clinicians, that is, continuing education and supervision (13); and articles related to medical students and other health professionals (24), which also evidenced the social work and health care connection.

The topics of collaboration and multidisciplinary team activities (70;10%) substantiated the social workers' biopsychosocial commitment to patient care in their partnerships with other health care professionals. In 58 (8.2%), the subjects of professional accountability and program evaluation were seen in the context of quality assurance (QA) and quality improvement (QI) and were therefore undertaken as studies of practice and programs. Changing health care was a topic in 53 (7.6%) publications and overlapped as a subject in many of the other categories. Performance, practice, management, QI, discharge planning, consumer education, program development, and ethics were affected by governmental, technological changes, and the educational advances social workers made. Changes in care delivery to patients and families are readily observed in the writings.

Thirty (4.3%) articles on management and administration reflected the service problems within the institution and emphasized the need to develop and introduce new programs. As consumers of care became more vocal, two areas captured the interest of social workers: community and lay participation (19; 2.7%) and consumer health education. Social workers at Mount Sinai began to write health education articles for the lay market in the 1970s, and their writings in this area increased exponentially in the 1980s, reaching a total of 48 articles (6.9%) by the end of 1991.

THE AUTHORS' VIEW

Practitioners developed this review, and their observations and analyses of the writings thus might reflect an approach biased toward practice, based on awareness of the "art of practice" and on belief in the value and benefits of direct social services. Social work practitioners are critical in the health care of individuals and must function as partners with other health care professionals, the medical institution, and the community. For the clinician, the client is an adventure, a mystery in which the past and the present must be unraveled as the clinician pursues a one-on-one, a group, or a community relationship. Working directly with clients, the clinician is *in* and *with* the process and not merely an observer of it. A clinical practice by qualified social workers leads to change in performance both in social work and institutional programs as well as change in a vast array of indirect functions that benefit people.

In analyzing the published works by decade and by specific topic area, we hoped to reflect on the trends in social work in health care over a 40-year period. Responses to clients, the community, and the organization are evidenced and result in a prescription for social work in health care today and tomorrow. We believe that what follows clearly illustrates the phenomenal progress social work practitioners have made in four decades and the societal context in which the powerful challenges of the future of social work lie.

2

Health Care and the Social Work Connection

Helen Rehr

EARLY HISTORY

To view the history of social services in the United States in the context of health care requires a look at the early stages of lay charity services for the sick at home and in a range of institutions. In the United States and England, the hospital of the 18th century was an almshouse, an all-purpose social welfare institution with no remedial services. Social services and hospitals have their beginnings in the United States in the late 19th and early 20th centuries. However, ministration to the "sick poor" has existed in one form or another and has been noted since the beginning of recorded history. Experiences were recorded in the Middle East at Damascus, Baghdad, and Alexandria. In Spain the Saracens founded hospitals of opulent luxury, which the Crusaders used as examples when they returned home, opening medical care institutions with a social service overlay for the sick poor.

To establish the historical beginnings of social work is to perhaps credit (St.) Vincent de Paul "as the patron saint of all hospital social services" (MacKenzie, 1919). The formal beginnings of medically focused social services conceivably began in 1636 with his ministrations. From then until the French Revolution, Parisian hospitals had full-fledged social service auxiliaries whose functions included soliciting and contributing funds, visiting ward patients, and visiting discharged patients in their homes. They paralleled today's workers—as fundraisers seeking essential financial support, as visitors who brought "material and moral aid" to those on the wards, and as home visitors; informed by the ward aides about individual case requirements, they advised, directed, and assisted convalescents.

The system was abandoned during the French Revolution but reestablished after the revolution first as a Hotel de Dieu, the French term for the resting place where the terminally ill would get ready to "meet their Maker." Soon hospitals were reformulated, and each had a type of social service auxiliary.

St. Vincent de Paul's work was prompted by both religious and humanitarian motives; the chief beneficiaries in France were Roman Catholics. An organization was created under Protestant auspices in 1867 (Goldwater, 1919). Sir William Blizzard is credited with a comparable organized effort on behalf of the sick poor in the development of the London Hospital in 1791. Shortly after the London Charity Organization Society (the Society) was created in 1869 to improve conditions of the poor and repress mendacity a great protest arose from doctors who had organized against the abuse of "free care" in clinics by those who could and should pay a private fee. In 1874 the Royal Free Hospital asked the Society to determine the social position of a group of outpatients in an attempt to exclude those ineligible for free care. Charles Loch suggested the need for a 'charity assessor' (the hospital almoner to be) to handle financial-eligibility screening. Patients in need were referred to the Society. Those who could pay a small fee were referred to Provident Dispensaries, fixed-fee clinics set up to manage the abuse problem.

The English hospital almoner was formally recognized in 1895 when for the first time an experienced social worker from the Society was stationed at The Royal Free Hospital "to review applicants for admission to the dispensary and to exclude those unsuitable for free care" (Cannon, 1952). Thus one of the first roles of medical social service workers in England was to screen and exclude those who could pay for private medical care. Later, as these almoners screened for eligibility, they began to identify other social needs related to welfare relief and illness. The National Health Insurance Act of 1911 broadened the scope of the almoners' social services.

IN THE UNITED STATES

The formal beginning of medical social work services for the sick in this country occurred more than 200 years after the work of St. Vincent de Paul.

The eighteenth and early nineteenth century history of nursing and medical care was glaringly black, with only small pockets of innovation occurring among the medical and social leaders of the different periods (Deutsch, 1946). The proprietary type of medical institution was indigenous to the New World, where unprecedented rapid expansion of population over enormous territory created a demand for doctors long before facilities existed for their training. Conditions in these institutions were chaotic. The pioneering conditions of the country produced thousands of doctors with little knowledge and skill, trained in commercial medical schools established for profit. Hospitals established by municipalities, religious organizations, and philanthropic groups were also apprenticeship locales for doctors-in-training (Flexner, 1925).

Social and environmental conditions in the mid-19th century were appalling as the United States shifted from an agrarian to an urban society. As the Northeast became industrialized and urbanized it supported increasing waves of immigrants who worked as unskilled laborers in sweatshop factories and lived in slums. Disease was rampant, food and housing conditions were primitive, and poverty was everywhere (Rosenberg, 1967). Early in the 19th century, pauperism was considered inherited; by the end of the 1800s, rugged individualism—the Social Darwinian concept of survival of the fittest—had surfaced as a popular belief. A strong work ethic was prevalent and social morality was considered a key virtue. Both were believed essential in the poor if they were to improve their status. The pattern of the times was to remove the unfit from the community (Axinn & Levin, 1975), and welfare generally was custodial rather than remedial.

Medicine and social work crawled into the 20th century with no organized base, although they supported the Darwinian beliefs. Medicine had no scientific base and its ministrations had little therapeutic benefit. Rich and poor alike avoided American doctors and hospitals. In Europe, however, new discoveries, new understandings of disease, and new techniques were developing. This scientific knowledge was transmigrated at the turn of the century to those American medical establishments affiliated with universities (Rosner, 1978).

Social-environmental issues of this period included a depression, economic uncertainty, massive immigration from all parts of Europe, development of a new capitalist class, and a growing labor class. These social-environmental factors were reflected in growing patterns of illness, disease, and disability and may have contributed to the changing character of medicine. They certainly affected social welfare: rampant social breakdown resulted in the rise of a social reform movement fostered by social work's early leaders and socially minded citizens (Leiby, 1978).

WOMEN AND THE SICK

Women were the primary caretakers of the sick poor; whether in the early hostels or in latter-day hospitals, they have remained at the forefront of direct and indirect service through ladies aid societies and/or auxiliaries. As observers they reported on conditions. As providers of services they were the first hospital "social service" workers, visiting patients in the hospital and patients and families in their homes, where they helped secure compliance with medical recommendations using whatever mechanisms were known. They emphasized environmental and material needs.

It was these pioneering volunteer women who brought a social and humane orientation to medical institutions (MacEachern, 1940). The social services in American hospitals, formally initiated in 1905 at Massachusetts General Hospital, evolved from the work of lay women who facilitated development of organized social services and nursing by prodding the male-dominated medical institutions to respond to the social needs of the poor. The women of Mount Sinai are part of that history via an auxiliary board whose objective was "to supplement the medical care provided by the hospital with such services as will further the welfare of the patient and his family" (Stein, undated). In addition to its continuing support of social services, the auxiliary board initiated a host of programs that were institutionalized and professionalized over time—the volunteer program, occupational therapy, diversional and recreational services, a patient's library, a play school and kindergarten, job training and a sheltered workshop, rehabilitation, convalescent and camp care supports, home care, speech therapy, and services to aid neighboring community residents, as well as support for many interdisciplinary social-health programs.

Women in medicine tended to remain in the background. But at Mount Sinai in the 1870s, farsighted male leaders of the newly created medical board (Drs. Abraham Jacobi, Samuel Percy, and Charles Budd) persuaded the other male trustees, who originally rejected women physicians in the hospital, to employ women physicians to serve on female wards.

Women in nursing did not face these obstacles in the locus of service, although they were viewed merely as physicians' handmaidens and patient aides. Florence Nightingale's exposure of hospitals as deathtraps was followed by her pioneering efforts in nursing education. She was responsible for the early focus on quality hospital care and she introduced bedside teaching. Her basic philosophy taught that one nursed the sick and not the sickness (Lyons & Petrucelli, 1978; p. 547). It took a long time for that philosophy to become a focus of medical care, and it is still absent in some areas of health services. Over time, nurses have been influential in enhancing medical care and in initiating social services in medical settings.

MEDICAL EDUCATION AND SOCIAL SERVICES

Physicians—such as Adolph Meyer, Richard Cabot, William Osler, Francis Peabody, and Charles Emerson—created the aftercare movement in psychiatry with nurses and lay leaders. In this program, the social worker acted as investigator and information gatherer for these doctors, who acknowledged that social and environmental factors were responsible for certain diseases. Their beliefs led to development of supports in the form of home care and social services to ambulatory patients in mental health clinics, and to families. These leaders brought to medical education the concept of exposing their students to the community environment, to people's working conditions, and to their homes in order to determine the etiology of illnesses. Medical students worked with the new medical social service workers as "friendly visitors." Both medicine and social work adopted a hands-on approach to field education that emphasized the family, the neighborhood, and the workplace.

SOCIAL REFORM AND THE SOCIAL SERVICES

The charity organization and the settlement house movements revealed the vast social and health needs of people living in crowded, deplorable urban conditions. Prevention and improvement of the social-health of individuals arose as the means to address social problems. This led to a social reform movement directed at legislatures and communities, led by the leading social reformers of the era—Dorothea Dix, Jane Addams, and Edith Abbott (Axinn & Levin, 1975; p. 99), who were joined by physicians who held similar beliefs. At the direct service level, social services were established on behalf of sick children with an emphasis on strengthening "at home" needs of mothers in the care of their children.

One outcome of the social reform movement was that social services, like medicine and later nursing, separated the clinical role from social welfare and also from public health. All three professions moved to claim the clinical in the care of the individual as their primary function, with social-health policy as secondary; and this separation still exists today. At the turn of the century, however, Mount Sinai leaders joined with others in initiatives directed at both direct services and social-health concerns, specifically tuberculosis, by securing the establishment of sanatoria in New York State as early as 1904, and by promulgating mental health reforms. In 1906 a philanthropically supported social welfare department was created and by 1908 the hospital noted the permanent budgetary support of social services. "It is now recognized that the condition of a patient's family while he is in our wards, as well as his needs immediately after his discharge from the hospital, constitute so vital a part of his ability to re-cover, and to retain his health, that the work of this department has come to be recognized as a legitimate part of the functions of this institution" (Hirsch & Doherty, 1952; p. 151).

In performing their services, social workers frequently were directed by the expectations of bureaucrats or physicians. Issues of control of the who, what, how, and when of social work responsibility were not always the primary aegis of social workers who, like nurses, frequently were re-ferred to as physicians' handmaidens. Both nursing and social work, which were female-dominated, had to find ways "to control their perfor-mance," seeking autonomy (Friedson, 1970; p. 88). The issue of profes-sional autonomy versus administrative authority is still common. Along with interprofessional conflicts, the issue surfaces again and again in many forms. Turf conflicts are still prevalent between doctor and nurse, doctor and social worker, nurse and social worker, social worker and hospital ad-ministrator, and between those dual authorities responsible for institu-tional service: the medical and lay boards. Roles and functions have become confused, and they overlap.

THE EVOLUTION OF SOCIAL WELFARE BENEFITS

The Roosevelt Administration had first promulgated the right to medical care in the form of a national health insurance program, which was debated but not achieved. The Social Security Act of 1935, which created many so-cial welfare benefits, was expanded in 1965 to include health care costs for the elderly (Medicare), and the needy poor (Medicaid), and an expanded maternal and child health service, including services to disabled children. Concurrent with health care payment programs by federal and state gov-ernments, a burst of new advanced medical technologies changed the hos-pital and health care system and resulted in today's "health care industry."

In the social work emphases of the 1940s a major shift began from psy-choanalytic theory, which dominated social services from World War I to World War II, to the influence of the social sciences, which were beginning to achieve status and recognition. Social workers again integrated a broad social concern into their philosophy. The neighborhood and community were seen as venues for services for individuals and groups at-risk. Group services and community development efforts were introduced, and their beginnings are observed in social work services in health care settings.

In the 1950s and 1960s, although fiscal concerns surfaced periodically, a burst of affluence resulted in major social and health care change. The civil rights movement, the women's movement, the drug culture, and the sexual revolution took their places in history as instigators of sea change in social mores. More technological initiatives were introduced than in the entire previous history. An explosion of federalism occurred in the medical and social work fields, including the Hill-Burton Act for the construction of hospital beds; an expanded Public Health Service; a burgeoning Veterans' Administration; the Health Professions' Education Act; Medicare, Medicaid, and the Maternal and Child Health Programs; and active support of biomedical research in the field by the National Institutes of Health. Innovative services for veterans and for handicapped children took hold. Rehabilitation, developed by Dr. Howard Rusk during World War II, flourished as physical medicine become the preferred treatment for the growing numbers of disabled adults and children. Poliomyelitis, the scourge of the 1960s, adopted rehabilitation as a significant treatment modality. The recognition that parents were essential care providers for children with chronic illnesses influenced the origins of family therapy, extended to the treatment of the mentally ill.

Many of the benefits of the 1950s and 1960s are fast being constricted as a result of fiscal crises and a taxpayers' revolt that furthered conservatism in limiting the support of existing social benefits and resulted in a major change in social policy. In health policy, the national focus in the 1970s, 1980s, and 1990s shifted from a commitment of governmental efforts to assure high-quality, comprehensive care, to a so-called safety net, to capped limits in medical care that resulted in fewer services for the needy (Rehr & Rosenberg, 1986; p. 80). In the 1990s, although millions more are being served in hospitals across the country, the major cities have been dramatically affected by the large number of homeless persons and illegal aliens, sick without insurance, and a significant aging population making large demands on the health care system's resources. Life styles are different, and more diversity exists in communities than homogeneity. The work environment is changing constantly, affected by new technology that directly affects workers in the workplace and also their health status. The national fiscal crisis has resulted in newly unemployed skilled and professional workers.

From 1980 to today, health care has been reshaped, and responsibility for payment of services falls more and more to the individual. Increased premiums, larger deductibles, cutbacks by the federal government in all its programs and to the states for their services, and curtailed employee health benefit programs have meant more out-of-pocket costs for everyone and precipitated lack of coverage or limited insurance for between 35 and 60 million Americans. These are persons with marginal incomes, including Blacks and Hispanics, those in uncovered work situations, millions of children of the marginally employed, the poor over 65 years of age, and the homeless.

The fiscal crisis affected hospitals as early as the mid-1970s when they were expected to monitor patient utilization of services. The shift from per diem reimbursement for length-of-stay to diagnosis-related groups (DRGs) changed the pattern of care from hospital inpatient services irrespective of length of stay to prescheduled hospitalization and greater emphasis on ambulatory services.

Deregulation of health care, a 1980s phenomenon, changed the health care system from a public social utility and voluntary care system to commercialized medical care. For-profit health enterprises entered the marketplace, adding a third tier of care to that of the voluntary and public hospitals. Traditional charitable support for these hospitals had been incorporated into a charitable cost factor in the reimbursement provided by third-party payers. With privatization of hospitals came a practice of "skimming" the private or well-insured patients, who generally were less ill than the medically indigent. This practice resulted in cost benefits to for-profit hospitals and in turn to severe fiscal damage to voluntary and municipal hospitals.

Federal and state governments capped their reimbursement levels, and de facto rationing of care became commonplace. Not only were benefits and services changed, but beds (and hospitals) were closed when occupancy rates were considered too low to support them. In general, bed-occupancy rates hovered at 60% in the 1980s. An empty bed remains a cost factor because services such as staff and maintenance must be continued. Unfortunately, the AIDS epidemic caused a lack of availability of beds to this population and a shortfall of acute and long-term care.

The introduction of DRGs affected the average length-of-stay as well as the number of hospital admissions. It also caused a major increase in ambulatory visits. Voluntary and municipal hospitals now serve a greater concentration of sicker in-hospital persons, which places heavier demands on health care providers in contrast to the previous case mix of the sick and less sick. Whether those who have been seriously ill are discharged prematurely or not, more people leave the hospital in need of at-home support services, which are limited even for those who can afford them. Shortened hospital stays might reduce the cost of hospitalization but not the overall cost of illness, which rises because of other factors. Additional costs of direct services at-home can affect discharged patients as do the indirect social costs to their family members of patient care at-home (Ancona-Berk & Chalmers, 1986).

DRGs have precipitated at least one major social benefit: discharged patients return earlier to familiar surroundings that generally are more supportive than hospital surroundings (Simon *et al.*, 1995). Social work has played an increasing role in early discharge planning and in securing optimum "assists" for patients and families. Because health care requires a continuum that goes beyond the walls of the hospital and the offices of doctors, health care social workers must learn to function outside of the institution.

The changing health care delivery system and payment environment require redefinition of roles and functions. Linkages with voluntary and private community support services are being negotiated, and in-house and at-home rehabilitation, both in physical and social functioning, are projected for early intervention. Not-for-profit medical institutions have begun to compete with for-profit institutions. The falling occupancy rate, cutbacks in reimbursement, and the impact on revenues have transformed the more enterprising medical institutions into market-driven enterprises that focus on wellness and fitness programs, behavioral medicine, drug and alcohol abuse, and eating disorders. Emphasis on a "one-stop shopping" focus for a specific chronic illness is a burgeoning direction. Chronic illnesses and disabilities are treated in multiservice centers. Specialty services are in vogue, such as those that focus on the social-health needs of women and children and cover both medical and social services, including counseling modalities and health education and maintenance. Programs are staffed by many disciplines as growing interdependence among health care professionals occurs.

The academic medical centers continue to either create or join in community/regional public health endeavors with consumers and potential consumers of care to address the current needs of sick individuals and families (Melum, 1989) as well as social and political health care issues. Health education and prevention programs are being introduced into communities with the help of local residents. Partnership between hospital providers and consumers is more evident than ever before. Diversification and new organizational approaches emphasize wellness; today's children are tomorrow's adults and will live an average of 80 years in the community. Reduced government support for these community-based enterprises, however, will take its toll.

Managed care programs have proliferated. Many are commercial enterprises with a cost-containment rather than quality-of-care focus. Although industry has sought managed care programs to control utilization of services, concern is mounting about their lack of measurement of quality, superimposed costs, and occasional denial of professionally determined services. In addition, managed care companies have not provided for the uninsured nor focused on public health. However, if quality of care is a component of service, then cost-containment through managed care must be relevant in the context of cost-effective service.

Downsizing, commonplace in corporate America, is occurring in health care institutions which face lower occupancy rates, changed reimbursement patterns, and major shifts from inpatient to ambulatory care, particularly same-day surgery and new technological services. Many hospitals have expanded their ambulatory services, linked with physician group practices, and merged or affiliated with other medical institutions to secure traffic flow and cost savings. With downsizing has come reengineering of inpatient services; to achieve purported cost savings, institutions have created patient-centered care units using trained in-house personnel.

SOCIAL WORK SERVICES IN THIS CENTURY

Social work services were formalized in the United States in 1905 when Richard Cabot recognized their importance to his patients. By the mid-1920s, Flexner (1915) had studied social work, identified its many problems, and attempted to formalize a scientific base to its services. Mary Richmond (1917) had written *Social Diagnosis*, and social workers were attempting to integrate social diagnoses into medical diagnoses. Social and environmental conditions were recognized as contributors to diseases. By the late 1920s and early 1930s, social work moved to accept a psychoanalytic framework for its casework services. The Great Depression confirmed the need for a range of welfare benefits and concrete services that also were delivered by government and agency-based social services.

The major shift toward recognizing formal social work services began during World War II as social mores changed. Other shifts took place as new technology advanced, fiscal crises occurred, and hospital lengths-of-stay were shortened. Social workers brought new emphasis to their changing roles, practicing in new venues and expanding their purview. As practice skills were advanced, social workers recognized the transitional patterns of illness and disability. When chronic disorders became the majority, social work concentration shifted to a concept of functional limitations and individual and family strengths. While disease and disability were critical, it was in working with the individual and family network that some level of quality-of-life could be achieved—striving for optimal social and physical functioning within a rehabilitative context in the individual's social environment, a shift to a social-health focus.

Clinical skills and models of care advanced. Family-focused counseling, support groups for patients and/or family members, and psychoeducational programs were introduced. Social workers recognized the need to develop partnerships with their clients to achieve mutually shared treatment goals and to identify each other's responsibilities, the basis for treatment contracts (client/provider partnerships) which were a source of outcome study information. Problem classification delineation and outcome/patient satisfaction studies were tools to determine the impact of care on patients and whether new services and programs and/or improved performance and care were necessary.

The introduction of high social-risk screening facilitated other social epidemiological approaches. As social workers aggregated client situations, differences in subgroup populations became apparent. Cultural diversity was recognized, and new knowledge about the influence of culture on social-health issues developed. Social workers also learned general clinical variables relevant to given groups, which permitted early and enhanced assessment of individual social-health problems; that is, workers were able to apply subgroup variables to individual client situations. Social workers enhanced their collaboration with other health care professionals, contributing not only to diagnosis and treatment but also to joint program evaluation. Providing consultation to physicians, institutional administrators, and community-based social workers often was expected.

Shared treatment goals with patients focused on a continuum of care, often extending to the home for long-term aftercare. The patient and both informal and formal networks were involved; follow-up became commonplace. The venues of care began to shift, and social workers met their clients in doctors' offices and in newly established outpatient services. Managed care concentrated on capping ambulatory and inpatient care, making brevity in services essential.

As they encountered barriers to and fragmentation of care for their clients, social workers took on new roles, including patient representation and social-health advocacy. These programs began to socialize the institution to individualized patient care; others concentrated on encouraging administration to shift from a staff focus to patient needs as a primary responsibility. Employee assistance programs that focused on social-health problems also were introduced.

The fiscal crisis in health care delivery placed a new emphasis on social work. Just as 19th century social workers were expected to exclude paying clients from service, today's social workers are expected to produce revenue either directly or indirectly. This affirms the changed pattern of social services for marginal and low- income people to include those who can afford to pay for social services either personally or through insurance. Social workers have reached out into the community to find those in need of social-health care, and to encourage their use of the institution, enhancing the revenue base.

These new social work functions and roles are the result of an aggressive social work leadership which recognized that leadership responsibilities are not limited to clients served, but extend to an institution's clientele, its communities, and the public in general. Many social work leaders have been appointed to and serve administrative functions within institutions while maintaining their roles as social workers and providing individual client services.

CONCLUSION

"No institution is separate from its times. It either is in the vanguard or it lags behind, and in most cases both patterns exist with more of one and less of the other. The responses to demand, and the pulls of personal and professional expectations are those of the leaders in the institution and in the broader arena" (Rehr, 1982).

We have briefly placed social work in health care in the context of social change and institutional change. Social workers in health care settings are no longer handmaidens to doctors. Theirs is a new relationship within the institution and with other health care providers as they initiate and implement social-health services. They emphasize their professional independence while they enter into sound collaborative and team relationships.

The history of social work tells us what has been tried, under what conditions, and what has prevailed. The language of the past and present is similar, but the changes in social, scientific, and technological areas are tremendous. These changes have created a different terrain over which social workers, their health care partners, and their clientele will travel. Social work in health care looks ahead to the innovative planning of health care security for everyone, guaranteeing individuals and communities access to basic health services.

MOUNT SINAI REFERENCES

HEALTH CARE AND THE SOCIAL WORK CONNECTION

1950s

Siegel D (1957). Social work in the medical setting: An instrument for health. *Social Work*, April:70–77.
Steinberg M, Siegel D (1956). The medical social service—necessity or luxury? *Hospitals*, March, reprint.

1960s

Dana B (1969). Social work in the university medical center. *The Johns Hopkins Medical Journal*, 124(5):277–282.

Siegel D (1962). Changing character of the Jewish hospital: Implications for social service administration. *Journal of Jewish Communal Services, 38*(3):282–289.

Zousmer G (1967). Social work and social agencies: Contribution to medical practice. *Medical Clinics of North America, 51*(6):1485–1491.

1970s

Berkman B (1977). Community mental health services for the elderly. *Community Mental Health Review, 2*(3):1–9.

Dana B (1973). Health and social work and social justice. *Social Practice and Social Justice.* Monograph. Washington DC: National Association of Social Workers, Inc., 111–128.

Lurie A, Rosenberg G (Eds.). (1977). *Social Work in Mental Health: A 25 Year Perspective.* New Hyde Park, NY: L.I. Jewish Hospital Medical Center.

Lurie A, Rosenberg G, Ron, HZ (1977). Governmental processes influencing mental health. In A Lurie, G Rosenberg (Eds.). *Social Work in Mental Health.* New Hyde Park, NY: L.I. Jewish Medical Center, *VIII*:62–75.

Siegel D, Rehr H (1971). Evolving social services in psychiatry. *The Mount Sinai Journal of Medicine, 38*(2):185–197.

Young AT (1974). Contemporary woman and her family: Implications for social work program and practice in obstetrics and gynecology. *The Proceedings of the First National Workshop on the Delivery of Hospital Social Work Services in Obstetrics and Gynecology and Services to the Newborn.* New Haven, CT: Yale-New Haven Medical Center, DHEW Publ. #77-5026:77–80.

1980s

Clarke S (1983). Hyman J. Weiner's use of systems and population approaches: Their relevance to social work practice today. *Social Work in Health Care, 9*(2):5–14.

Lewis M (1982). Aging in the people's republic of China. *International Journal of Aging and Human Development, 5*(2):79–105.

Miller R, Rehr H (Eds.). (1983). *Social Work Issues in Health Care,* Englewood Cliffs, NJ: Prentice-Hall.

Rehr H (Ed.). (1982). *Milestones in Social Work and Medicine: Social-Health Care Concepts.* New York: Prodist.

Rehr H (1982). Social work and medicine at Mount Sinai: Then and now. In H Rehr (Ed.). *Milestones in Social Work and Medicine: Social-Health Care Concepts.* New York: Prodist:42–59.

Rehr H (1982). More Thoughts on American Health Care. In H. Rehr (Ed.). *Milestones in Social Work and Medicine: Social-health Care Concepts.* New York: Prodist:83–104.

Rehr H (1985). Medical organization and the social service connection: Past, present and future. *Health and Social Work, 10*(4):245–257.

Rosenberg G, Grace N (1982). Group services and medical illness. In A Lurie, G Rosenberg, and S Pinsky (Eds.). *Social Work with Groups in Health Settings.* New York: Prodist:39–53.

Young AT (1989). Strengths of families: Past, present and future. *Proceedings on Empowering Families for Better Health, Maternal and Child Health and Resources Development.* U.S. Public Health Service and University of South Carolina, Columbus.

3

Clinical Interventions and Social Work Roles and Functions

Helen Rehr, Gary Rosenberg, and Susan Blumenfield

The social work profession encompasses multiple roles and functions; knowledge, values, and skills underpin almost all aspects of social work engagement. The skills required for clinical intervention with consumers of services are similar to those required in working with health care providers, individuals in programs and planning, administrators, regulators, and community groups. Social workers in health settings bring a person or family-centered model of care to assessment and treatment, which differs from the patient-focused medical model.

Although additional knowledge and skills might be essential to ensure quality performance in the broader multidisciplinary arena of social-health services, social work's basic values and ethics prevail. They are predicated on recognizing the patient's dignity, worth, and need to seek self-determination as well as on recognizing one's own values and the need to protect the patient from harm. Knowledge and values are implemented successfully in health care at the interface between clients and providers when expectations are mutually agreed upon, and when institutional and community social systems are flexible enough to allow modifications that enhance services and their quality when necessary.

It is within the framework of values and ethics that the clinical interventions and social work roles and functions developed and applied over a period of almost 40 years are reviewed. We believe that this framework is the foundation of all aspects of social work engagement, including program development, management and administration, quality improvement (applied studies), health education and prevention, community and lay participation, and lay and professional relationships. The evidence of knowledge and values permeates them, and interventive skills affect both program and practice.

SOCIAL WORK IN HEALTH CARE

Social workers in health settings integrate a person/family-oriented, biopsychosocial model of care into their practice as they strive to identify the needs of sick patients and their families. They recognize that informal support systems (e.g., those provided by family) as well as formal supports (e.g., those provided in a community) are essential in facilitating the quality of life of the sick and disabled. The setting in which social workers practice also is critical, in that it can either enhance or impede the quality of services. Health policies, legislation, institutional programs, and an individual's cultural and environmental background and life-style patterns are key factors that affect how the client and social worker meet and work together.

No field or discipline can encompass all that is known to date about health and illness. However, all disciplines know that in illness a biological alteration affects both the physical and social status of individuals, who experience their illness based on cultural, economic, educational, psychological, and social factors. Social workers in health settings must be knowledgeable about disease, disability, and mental illness. The social work profession has been successful in integrating a biopsychosocial construct in its work with patients and families, which has been fundamental in the profession's collaboration with physicians and other health care professionals and which has led to a shift in medicine from a biomedical to a biopsychosocial orientation.

As social workers perceived needs, new programs were projected to match the needs, frequently through a specific clinical intervention such as family therapy, group therapy, crisis intervention, or psychoeducation. As clinical interventions are applied, their outcomes must be evaluated. In most instances, practitioners require new knowledge as they reach toward new ways to serve clients. Such knowledge usually is achieved though experience and/or study of existing services. Edward Kilborne (1986) suggests that observation leads us to question and study, which can result in change. Clinical activity and observed experiences result in more knowledge about sickness, its patterns and treatments, health maintenance, individual and family attitudes and behaviors, the setting in which services take place, and how to ensure successful collaboration with other health care professionals. Ethical dilemmas are not uncommon in a complex organization in which one works with other health care colleagues or hospital administrators. When examined, any differences among workers can lead to changes in program and/or practice.

THE RELEVANT LITERATURE

In the 1950s, the practice of medicine focused primarily on the biological and anatomical, and social work was viewed as a luxury. Social work publications from that period reflect the belief that it was essential to socialize administrators and health care professionals to the necessity of social services. Doctors and administrators believed they knew what was best for patients and so informed them. Medical care was unilinear (i.e., from doctors to patients, who had a passive relationship with the medical establishment).

COMPREHENSIVE, CONTINUOUS CARE

Social work broadened care from environmental task functions and demonstrated that psychosocial-environmental components affected diagnosis and treatment and the manner in which people handled medical advice. Social workers observed that people with chronic illnesses needed comprehensive, coordinated care that continued into the home after discharge. The poliomyelitis epidemic helped social workers understand how patients' body image affected recovery. Building a positive self-image through a rehabilitation focus could not be limited to physical deficits but had to focus on psychological and social components as well. The recognition that continuity of care after discharge was essential led to new concepts about physical and spatial relationships in rehabilitation directed toward helping the patient achieve optimum physical function. Social workers also recognized that counseling about body image and gains in social functioning were critical to achieving any form of physical restoration. Moreover, counseling families and expanding their knowledge about the disease and expectations for the patient were critical to strengthening families' ability to support patients and help their motivation and sense of self.

Although poliomyelitis was one of the first, other chronic illnesses raised the same issues, and the common dimensions of chronic illnesses were recognized. Additional comprehensive programs were developed as social workers became more specialized and established new roles in the treatment of rheumatic disease, hemophilia, chronic obstructive pulmonary disease (COPD), amyotrophic lateral sclerosis (ALS), neurofibromatosis, and cancer, among others. The need for family therapy became a common denominator in all chronic disease, helping both patients and families face the complexity of care with professional guidance. Social workers created specialized care programs for children and adolescents and for the parents of those children; that is, support groups for chronically ill children and their parents. The ongoing needs of the chronically ill, in particular the elderly, required use of available community resources to offer formal supports where needed. Networking took hold and linkages among service organizations became essential for cost-effective care and for continuity of care. These social work endeavors continue into the present, modified by new knowledge, new experiences, and new social workers.

In both adult and children's psychiatric services, the concept of comprehensive care for schizophrenics and other mentally disordered patients was translated into a psychoeducational function that trains patients and families to draw on positive behaviors and situational demands. At the same time, milieu and drug therapies have proved successful in certain situations. As new diseases were identified and became concerns of the medical care establishment, they also became critical social work service arenas. AIDS, a disease that affects such large numbers, required development of specific comprehensive care services. Again, social workers' past experiences with chronic illnesses facilitated development of services, although the bias, ostracism, and self-image and resource limitations of the disease required special focus. As substance abusers were drawn into social-health care, differences in ethnicity, gender, and class were considered because they appear to affect the way people reach out and respond to services.

PRENATAL CARE

In the 1950s, obstetrical services were concerned about the large numbers of unmarried mothers. Resource availability appeared directly related to how babies of unwed mothers would be cared for. Today, one of the major social-health concerns is pregnant women with AIDS and their newborns with HIV disease. Although in earlier decades social services focused on care of the infant and support of the mother, a range of health education, self-care, and support and community assistance programs have been introduced for prenatal women.

CONFRONTING TERMINAL ILLNESS

Changing attitudes toward the terminally ill brought new attention to dying patients. Doctors' attitudes toward informing patients about the diagnosis of terminal illness began to take on a new reality during the late 1970s and early 1980s, whereas denial and false hope previously had cloaked the issue. The work of Kubler-Ross (1969) reformed the clinical directions as providers gained understanding of human psychological responses to impending death. Social workers worked to help terminally ill patients and families discuss dying openly and plan for the end of life.

HUMAN SEXUALITY

The clinical social work concentration expanded from strictly helping the sick to helping healthy older persons handle their ongoing sexual interests. As cultural biases and stereotyping were recognized and addressed, sexuality in the older person was and continues to be seen and written about as a normal practice. Debility, senility, and general deterioration as an expectation of "old age" are recognized as myths; aging is an expanding field of study and societal attitudes toward age are changing among youth and the aging population itself.

VALUES AND ETHICS

In all professions that engage in human encounters, a social contract commits the professional to serve the "public good" and reach those in need. Inherent in this held value is social justice that ensures equity and fairness in how we as citizens are treated (pro publico bono). Other values guide professional behavior and action; they are translated operationally into ethical patterns. Although values might be clear, frequently they do not translate into action without ethical ambiguities. That is, social workers might be clear about their values on behalf of the public good, but ethical ambiguities can arise when dealing "ad hominem." Self-awareness, flexibility, integrity, and experience are qualities that help professionals face ambiguity and address personal anxiety, a not-infrequent response to dilemma. Relevant social work values include belief:

- in the dignity and worth of the individual;
- that an individual can be helped to reach his/her full potential; and
- that individual self-determination requires the right to know and be informed.

An accepted social-health care policy holds additional values for social workers who believe that:

- health care is a universal right;
- access to care should be guaranteed;
- a consumer should have a choice in care;

- care is based on expectations of mutual sharing and an informed partnership between consumer and provider;
- care should guarantee confidentiality;
- professional accountability is to the consumer first; and
- care is predicated on a biopsychosocial model.

Ethical dilemmas in patient care exist whenever decision making is unclear. In today's health care environment such dilemmas surface constantly. Expectations in care can differ widely among patients, families, health providers, social scientists, theologians, and even jurists and politicians who become actors in the "what should be done?" conundrum. Social issues that require value determination abound and force ethical considerations. In practice, making decisions calls on values that translate into ethical behaviors. For example, practitioners, especially physicians, long have faced the ethical dilemma of how much to tell a terminally ill patient. Although social workers have been more open to confronting the dilemma, the medical profession has begun to recognize the benefits of sharing details of care directly with patients. Patients and families who are well informed can make choices. Ethical determinants, such as assuring confidentiality and privacy, are professional requirements.

In a multidisciplinary environment, differences among team members in their recommendations often create additional ethical dilemmas. Sometimes differences surface in turf conflicts (i.e., which profession will handle what function). Although values can be professionally determined, subjectivity invariably exists. A legal or ethics clinic consisting of members of a patient-focused multidisciplinary team can successfully discuss complexities of institutional care, availability (or lack) of entitlements, and ethical dilemmas. Through open discussion of attitudes and beliefs, the forum attempts to reach consensus resolution and influence provider decision making.

PRACTICE SKILLS

The practice of social work in health care has been lodged in three dimensions: crisis (both situational and transitional), short-term and episodic treatment, and long-term therapy. Prevention and health maintenance, with their many health education measures, have become significant services in the 1990s. Social workers begin with the problem presented by the client system. The problem will require interventive skills such as assessment, problem formulation, and goal projections; collaboration with other health care providers; a partnership between client and social worker to achieve expected goals and to determine the functions each will undertake toward that end; a selection from a range of treatment modalities appropriate to the client and the problem; and outcome evaluation, including determining consumer opinion and satisfaction with care as well as that of the provider. The clinician's approach is inductive and draws on an experiential and programmatic response to the contract between patient and provider. The approach frequently is atheoretical, but always reflective and followed by action. Social workers in health care are patient/family-centered in their work, while their medicine and nursing colleagues are patient-centered.

Through the years, as social workers assumed new roles and functions and eliminated some from their early years, their professional armamentarium has expanded and they have become more skilled. The one-on-one direct casework or counseling function has remained primary, but new knowledge about personality, biopsychosocial factors, interpersonal relationships, disease and disability, community and resource availability, prevention and health maintenance, institutional demands, and cultural, educational, economic, and environmental factors demand special skills from the caseworker. Family and group therapy became commonplace, the latter in disease-specific groups of patients and spousal groups, parents' groups, and children's groups. When bereavement is a factor, group programs are very supportive. Depending on need and client expectation, they can be time-limited and/or long-term.

SOCIAL-RISK SCREENING

As individuals were admitted to the hospital for care, preadmission by telephone and in-person and at-admission screening for social risk were introduced to begin planning for quality discharge care. High social-risk screening is an effective social work casefinding measure, and social workers no longer are dependent on referrals, which invariably were late in a patient's stay and made quality planning difficult. Risk screening has uncovered patient need and allows for referral to care. Patients and families benefit from early planned intervention.

Crisis intervention as defined by Rapaport (1967) was particularly relevant for social workers who encountered many of their clients facing trauma with stress and anxiety. They successfully helped patients develop effective coping mechanisms. Brief therapy became valued for its exploration of immediate past concerns to help understand the present in a time-limited approach, to deal with and resolve a core conflict or issue. In most therapies social workers generally are active, arrive at mutual agreement about the problem at hand, and are open to the treatment method and responsibility of the client and the therapist. Hospital-based social workers have begun to move beyond the institutional walls into the community where they work in schools with teachers to find children with problems. They have joined with community agencies to introduce preventive services through a range of health education measures.

THERAPEUTIC TOOLS

New therapeutic tools have helped social workers significantly in their work with individuals. Oral history-taking is an excellent life-review therapy for the elderly. Pictographs help in work with the deaf. Special forms and interpreters help social workers in work with non-English-speaking clients. The problem-oriented patient record organizes the assessment process. Information in the patient record, when openly used with the client, demonstrates its therapeutic value as clients respond dynamically to being better informed.

STAFF SUPPORT GROUPS

As they worked with patients who had severe and disabling illnesses, social workers recognized how they personally were affected by their patients' debility. They turned to their supervisors for discussion and created support groups for themselves to help address their reactions and improve client relations. They created and led support groups for health care colleagues. Open discussion of feelings helped participants recognize that empathy with clients can be positive. Social workers assumed the role of consulting with other health care professionals about the biopsychosocial components of patient care early (see Chapter 7). The multidisciplinary setting made such consultation essential, particularly to physicians.

ADVOCACY

Advocacy is defined as the "act of directly representing, defending, interviewing, supporting, or recommending a course of action on behalf of one or more individual groups or communities with the goal of securing or retaining social justice" (Mickelson, 1995; p. 95). The function of advocacy, originally a tool of social workers, was expanded in response to patients encountering obstacles to service within the institution. The patient representative program facilitated inpatient care. Both patient representatives and social workers promoted access to the institution through their community activities. They helped patients navigate the confusing world of fragmented and duplicative services. Social-health advocates helped patients secure entitlements by referring them to appropriate public services. And finally, social workers testified before subcommittees of Congress to present the social-health needs of clients in efforts to secure legislative and regulatory change.

DISCHARGE PLANNING

Discharge planning in a quality context is written about from its many dimensions. Discharge planning has been viewed from the perspective of cost-containment through the impact of DRGs, seeking alternate care plans, enhancing "at-home" arrangements, and experimenting with controlled, abbreviated stays and early planned discharge (see Chapter 6).

FEE-FOR-SERVICE PROGRAMS

Private fee-for-services were introduced when it was recognized that private patients also need social services. Fee-for-service programs were initiated at first for geriatric patients and their families and have expanded to others in need. In addition, attending physicians sought social work services for office patients when they recognized that patients' social-health problems impede motivation and compliance, and thus recovery. In many instances, counseling and support services have been instrumental in reducing the number of unnecessary visits to physicians, who can be more productive in their overall services. When the institution introduced primary care, social workers joined doctors and nurses as primary caregivers in new primary care programs.

CONCLUSION

Marketing has made social services visible and has helped open the service door to clients in need, irrespective of economic status. But it is evident that the social workers who created roles and functions over 40 years of evolving practice were innovative; they recognized that identified needs demand solutions. In advancing their knowledge and skills, social workers also recognized the need to go beyond the institutional walls into the community. Public policy and cost constraints placed limits on continuity of care, a social work value. Although social work in health care had been largely confined to the hospital setting, social workers have expanded into the ambulatory setting in a variety of locations and have networked with other community social-health agencies. Today's social work follow-up of patients in posthospital care patterns the action of social workers in the 1950s who followed their polio patients into the home. High social-risk studies led social workers to focus on populations at-risk, as they drew upon epidemiological principles for assessment and for individualizing social treatment. As they supported their practice with studies, social workers introduced new functions and programs, simultaneously translating these innovative directions into the education of social workers, medical students and others (see Chapter 10).

According to Doernhofer and McNamara (1997), it is the tempo of practice that is difficult now. The need to conceptualize and assess more quickly is all-important. Clinical skills are put on fast-forward as a sense of pragmatism becomes essential. Patients and families present with multiple problems, and it is necessary to establish priorities quickly and be realistic about what can be done. Engagement skills are needed: be honest with the family and enable them to work together to achieve solutions. On the other hand, the principle of self-direction must underpin intervention. Problem-solving might be initiated in the hospital, but it must move to the outpatient clinic or the community to continue. Working with community resources often is difficult, and requires compatible clinical skills in deciding how to mobilize and use limited systems for families with limitations.

In today's practice, strong advocacy skills are a must—set skills. Social work practice is a playing field between two goal posts—one of human development, the other of social policy development. One gets better and better at acquiring techniques and viewpoints, but basically the rules and expectations are the same regardless of field or setting. A skilled clinician (practitioner) is responsive to the wide diversity of people served. The main task for all social workers is to create new ways of working within the changing, financially oriented health care environment, while simultaneously preserving basic social work values, knowledge skills, and ethics (Doernhofer & McNamara, 1997).

MOUNT SINAI REFERENCES

CLINICAL INTERVENTIONS, SOCIAL WORK ROLES AND FUNCTIONS, AND ETHICS

1950s

Fike, N (1957). Social treatment of long-term dependency. *Social Work*, October 51–56.
Kozier A (1957). Casework with parents of children born with severe brain defects. *Social Casework*, April.

Safran B, Spiegel F (1956). Helping a mother face medical crisis in a child. *Journal of Jewish Communal Services, 33*:180–184.

Siegel D (1953). The function of consultation. *Symposium Proceedings*. Pittsburgh, PA: School of Social Work, University of Pittsburgh:181–198.

Steinberg M, Siegel D (1956). Medical social service—necessity or luxury? *Hospitals*, March.

White E (1957). Casework service in a polio respiratory center. *Social Casework*, March.

1960s

Allen RE (1962). A study of subjects discussed by elderly patients in group counseling. *Social Casework*, July.

Berkman B, Rehr H (1968–1969). *Effects of differential timing of social service intervention with the aged*. Monograph, New York: The Mount Sinai Medical Center.

Dana B (1969). Social work in the university medical center. *The John Hopkins Medical Journal, 124*:277–282.

Paneth J (1961). Medical social services in the extra-marital pregnancy. *Journal of Jewish Communal Services, 37*:(Spring):270–279.

Siegel D (1962). Changing character of the Jewish hospital: implications for social service administration. *Journal of Jewish Communal Services, 38*:282–289.

Stein FT, Siegel D (1966). Survey of tasks and functions of social workers in the health field, its implications and challenges. *Proceedings of the Second Conference for Social Workers in the Health Field. National Conference of Jewish Communical Services*. Washington, DC:May 14–18:87–92.

Sweet A, White E (1961). Social and functional rehabilitation of patients with severe poliomyelitis. *The Mount Sinai Journal of Medicine, 28*:366–280.

White E (1961). The role of the community in rehabilitation. *Social Casework*, July.

White E (1961). The body-image concept in rehabilitating severely handicapped patients. *Social Work, 6*(3):51–58.

1970s

Berkman B (1977). Innovations for delivery of social services in health care. In F Sobey (Ed.). *Changing Roles in Social Work Practice*. Philadelphia, PA: Temple University Press.

Dana B (1979). Health care: A social service. In R Shannon (Ed.). *Retrospect and Prospect*. Pittsburgh, PA: School of Social Work, University of Pittsburgh:9–20.

Garfield M, Morganthau J (1976). Sex talks between mothers and daughters. *Medical Aspects of Human Sexuality,10*:6–18.

Lipton H, Malter S (1971). The social worker as mediator on a hospital ward. In W Schwartz, SR Zalba (Eds.). *The Practice of Group Work*. New York:97–121.

Levy LP (1977). Services to parents of children in a psychiatric hospital. *Social Casework*, April: 204–213.

Lowe JI (1978). Quality assurance in dialysis: The role of the social worker. *Journal of Dialysis, 2*:43–53.

Lowe JI, Herranen M (1978). Conflict in teamwork: Understanding roles and relationships. *Social Work in Health Care, 3*(3):323–330.

Maglin A (1974). An overdose of prejudice. *Human Behavior*, November:13.

Maglin A (1974). Sex role differences in heroin addiction. *Social Casework*, March:160–167.

Maglin A (1975). Casework with pregnant women on methadone maintenance. *Social Casework, 56*:131–137.

Maglin A (1978). Alienation and therapeutic intervention. *Catalyst, 2.*

Maglin A (1978). Some perspectives on psychoanalysis. *Catalyst,1*(1):100–102.

Mailick MD (1979). The impact of severe illness on the individual and the family: An overview. In A Davidson, S Clarke (Eds.). *Social Work Health Care: A Handbook for Practice.* New York: Haworth Press:101–113.

Mandelbaum E (1984). The family medicine consultant—reframing the contribution of medical social work. *Family Systems Medicine, 2*:310–319.

Mervis P (1977). Talking about the unmentionable: A group approach for cancer patients. In E Prichard, *et al.* (Eds.). *Social Work with the Dying Patient and the Family.* New York: Columbia University Press:233–241.

Paneth J, Lipsky H (1979). Utilization review and social work's role. In H Rehr (Ed.). *Professional Accountability for Social Work Practice: A Search for Concepts and Guidelines.* New York: Prodist:27–47.

Rehr H (1979). Social work looks to the future of health. In M Shipsey, J Morse (Eds.). *Successful Social Living for Sensory Deprived Persons.* Monograph. Boston, MA: Mass. Eye and Ear Hospital:98–106.

Rosenberg G, Attinson L (1977). Attitudes toward mental illness in the working class. *Social Work in Health Care, 3*(1):77–86.

Sampson N (1972). Family therapy for the child with a communicative disorder. *Journal of Communication Disorders, 5*(2):205–211.

Wincott E (1976). Comprehensive mental health services in the comprehensive care of the hemophiliac. *Proceedings Mental Health Services in the Comprehensive Care of the Hemophiliac,* May.

Wincott E (1977). Psychosocial aspects of hemophilia: problems, prevention, treatment modalities, research, and future directions. *The Mount Sinai Journal of Medicine, 44*:438–455.

Young AT, Berkman B, Rehr H (1973). Women who seek abortions: A study. *Social Work, 18*:60–65.

Young AT, Berkman B, Rehr H (1975). Parental influence on pregnant adolescents. *Social Work, 20*:387–391.

1980s

Becker D, Blumenfield S, Gordon N (1984). Voices from the eighties and beyond: Reminiscences of nursing home residents. *Journal of Gerontological Social Work, 8*(1/2):81–97.

Bennett C (1983). Commentary on Laura Epstein's 'short term treatment in health settings: Issues, concepts, dilemmas. In G Rosenberg, H Rehr (Eds.). *Advancing Social Work in the Health Care Field.* New York: Haworth Press:102–105.

Bennett C, Beckerman N (1986). The drama of discharge: worker/supervisor perspectives. *Social Work in Health Care, 11*(3):1–12.

Bennett C (1988). A social worker comments: Some implications for social work practice in health care settings. *Social Work in Health Care, 13*(4):15–18.

Bennett C, Legon J, Zilberfein F (1989). The significance of empathy in current hospital-based practice. *Social Work in Health Care, 14*(2):27.

Bennett C (1984). Testing the value of written information for patients and families in discharge planning. *Social Work in Health Care, 9*(3):95–97.

Black RB (1989). Editorial: prenatal diagnosis and fetal loss: Psychosocial conse-
quences and professional responsibilities. *American Journal of Medical Genetics,*
35:586–587.
Black RB (1989). A 1 and 6 month follow-up of prenatal diagnosis patients who lost
pregnancies. *Prenatal Diagnosis, 9:*794–804.
Black RB, Weiss JA (1989). Genetic support groups in the development of compre-
hensive genetic services. *American Journal of Human Genetics, 45:*647–654.
Bloom J, Ansell P, Bloom M (1989). Detecting elder abuse: A guide for physicians.
Geriatrics, 44(6):40–44, 56.
Blumenfield S, Morrison B, Stroh J, Fizdale R (1981). The elderly and the social
health care continuum. *Mount Sinai Journal of Medicine, 48*(6):569–572.
Blumenfield S (1982). Understanding and responding to the terminal patient. *Res-
ident and Staff Physician,* February:21–24.
Blumenfield M, Blumenfield S (1982). Talking to the patient with terminal illness.
Medical Times, 110: (May):73–76.
Blumenfield S (1983). The hospital center and the aging: A challenge for the social
worker. In G Getzel, J Mellor (Eds.). *Gerontological Social Work Practice in Long-
term Care.* New York: Haworth Press:35–59.
Blumenfield S (1986). Psychological and social effects of rheumatic disease during
late life. *Clinical Rheumatology in Practice, 4*(1):5–10.
Blumenfield S, Rosenberg G (1988). Towards a network of social health services:
Redefining discharge planning and expanding the social work domain. *Social
Work in Health Care, 13*(4):31–48.
Cantor M, Rehr H, Trotz V (1981). Case management and family involvement.
Mount Sinai Journal of Medicine, 48(6):566–568.
Cincotta N (1980). Open dialogue: adolescence. *Association of Pediatric Social Work-
ers Newsletter, 9:*(Fall):1.
Cincotta N (1987). Open dialogue: The question of coping. *Association of Pediatric
Oncology Social Workers Newsletter, 7:*(Fall/Winter):1.
Cincotta N (1989). Quality of life: A family decision. In J Van Eys (Ed.). *Cancer in the
Very Young.* Springfield, IL: CC Thomas:63–73.
Clarke S, Neuwirth L, Bernstein R (1986). An expanded social work role in a uni-
versity hospital-based group practice: An Service provider, physician educator
and organizational consultant. *Social Work in Health Care, 11:*1–18.
Daniels M (1980). Social work practice and community health: A planning imple-
mentation model. *Social Work in Health Care, 6:*39–51.
Fine C (1988). Social work: Facilitating family caregiving. *Productive Aging News:
The Mount Sinai Medical Center,* May:5–6.
Gantt AB, Goldstein G, Ponsky S (1989). Family understanding of psychiatric ill-
ness. *Community Mental Health Journal, 25:*101–108.
Gruber T (1980). The pre-admission screening process. In DR Heacock (Ed.). *A
Psychodynamic Approach to Adolescent Psychiatry: The Mount Sinai Experience.*
New York: Marcel Dekker:15–23.
Gruber T (1980). Ensuring that the system serves the patient. In DR Heacock (Ed.).
A Psychodynamic Approach to Adolescent Psychiatry: The Mount Sinai Experience.
New York: Marcel Dekker:305–309.
Gruber T (1983). Commentary on Laura Epstein's 'short-term treatment in health
settings: Issues, concepts, dilemmas. In G Rosenberg, H Rehr (Eds.). *Advancing
Social Work Practice in the Health Care Field.* New York: Haworth Press:98–101.

Hellinger-Kaslic J, Silverton M (1981). The changing role of the primary therapist on a short-term child psychiatry inpatient unit. In L Hoffman (Ed.). *The Evaluation and Care of Seriously Disturbed Children and Their Families*. New York: Spectrum:43–51.

Katch M (1983). Commentary on Helen Northern's 'social work groups in health settings: Promises and problems. In G Rosenberg, H Rehr (Eds.). *Advancing Social Work Practice in the Health Care Field*. New York: Haworth Press:121–123.

Katch M, Zayas L (1989). Contracting with adolescents: An ego psychological approach. *Social Casework*, January:3–9.

Katch M (1989). Acting out adolescents: The engagement process. *Child and Adolescent Social Work*, January.

Kirschner C, Rosengarten L (1982). The skilled social work role in home care. *Social Work*, 27:527–530.

Kohn, I (1986). Counseling women who request sterilization: Psychodynamic issues and interventions. *Social Work in Health Care*,11:35–60.

Levy LP, Joyce P, List J (1987). Reconciliations with parents as a treatment goal for adolescents in an acute care psychiatric hospital. *Social Work in Health Care*, 13(1):1–21.

Lewis M, Butler RN (1984). Life review therapy: Putting memories to work in individual and group psychotherapy. In E Burnside (Ed.). *Working with Elderly: Group Process and Technique*. Monterey, CA: Wadsworth:50–59.

Lewis M (1989). Sexual problems in the elderly, I: The use and abuse of medication. *Geriatrics*, 44(3):61–77.

Lewis M (1989). Sexual problems in the elderly, II: Men's vs women's. Geriatric panel discussion. *Geriatrics*, 44(3):(March):78–86.

Lewis M (1988). Caregiving: An emerging health issue. *America Meets Australia: Alzheimer's Disease—Researching the Questions*. South Melbourne, Australia: Alzheimer's Disease and Related Disorders Society.

Lipsky H, Sherman F (1984). Case study k—the geriatric evaluation and treatment service. In SJ Brody, NA Persily (Eds.). *Hospital and the Aged*. Rockville, MD: Aspen Systems Corp:219–225.

Lurie A, Rosenberg G, Pinsky S (Eds.) (1982). *Social Work with Groups in Health Care Settings*. New York:Prodist.

Maglin A (1980). Methadone maintenance. In R Herink (Ed.). *The Psychotherapy Handbook*. New York:377–379.

Mailick M (1989). The short term treatment of depression of physically ill hospital patients. In K Davidson, S Clarke (Eds.). *Social Work in Health Care: A Handbook for Practice*. New York:401–413.

Masser I, Caroscio JT, Luloff PB (1983). The team approach to the care of patients with amyotrophic lateral sclerosis. In LI Charash, SG Wolf, JT Caroscio, PB Luloff, A Bender (Eds.). *Psychosocial Aspects of Muscular Dystrophy and Allied Diseases*. Springfield, IL: CC Thomas:159–166.

Mervis P (1983). Commentary on Helen Northen's 'social work groups in health settings: Promises and problems. In G Rosenberg, H Rehr (Eds.). *Advancing Social Work Practice in the Health Care Field*. New York: Haworth:124–128.

Miller RS, Rehr H (1983). Health settings and health providers. In RS Miller, H Rehr (Eds.). *Social Work Issues in Health Care*. Englewood Cliffs, NJ: Prentice-Hall:1–19.

Morrison B (1981). Ethnic factors in service delivery to aged blacks in nursing homes. Ethnicity: An Issue for Human Services in the 1980s. *Findings and Implications of Recent Research, Community Council of Greater New York*. 12–22.

Morrison B (1983). Socio-cultural dimensions: Nursing homes and the minority aged. In G Getzel, J Mellor (Eds.). *Gerontological Social Work Practice in Long-Term Care.* New York:Haworth Press:127–145.

Morrison B (1984). Physical health and the minority aged. In R McNeely, J Colon (Eds.). *Aging in Minority Groups.* Glenwood Springs, CO:Sage Press.

Pincus S, Poliandro E (1983). A somaticizing adolescent: An approach to evaluation and therapy. *Journal of Adolescent Health Care,* 4:174–177.

Poliandro E (1989). Men, women and work. A study of involvement in work and non-work areas of adult life. *Social Work Research and Abstracts,* 25:112.

Rehr H, Berkman B, Rosenberg G (1980). Screening for high social risk: Principles and problems. *Social Work,* 25:403–406.

Rehr H (1983). Posing the issues. In G Rosenberg, H Rehr (Eds.). *Advancing Social Work Practice in the Health Care Field.* New York: Haworth Press:1–10.

Rehr H, Rosenberg G (1986). Access to social health care: Implication for social work. In H Rehr (Ed.). *Access to Social-health Care: Who Shall Decide What?* Lexington, MA: Ginn Press:77–96.

Rehr H (1986). Social work in health care for the eighties. In B Berkman (Ed.). *Social Work in Health Care.* Lectures, MGH Institute of Health Professions. Boston, MA:MGH.

Rehr H (1986). Discharge planning: An ongoing function of quality care. *Quality Review Bulletin,* 12:47–50.

Rosenberg G (1983). Advancing social work practice in health care. In G Rosenberg, H Rehr (Eds.). *Advancing Social Work Practice in the Health Care Field.* New York: Haworth Press:147–156.

Rosenberg G (1983). Practice roles and functions of the health social worker. In R Miller, H Rehr (Eds.). *Social Work Issues in Health Care.* Englewood Cliffs, NJ: Prentice-Hall:121–180.

Rosenberg G, Neill G (1982). Group services and medical illness. In A Lurie, G Rosenberg, S Pinsky (Eds.). *Social Work with Groups in Health Settings.* New York: Prodist:39–53.

Rosenberg G (1985). Clinical social work in health settings. *Social Casework,* 66:437–438.

Rosengarten L (1980). Taking on a filial role to care for frail elderly. *Practice Digest: A Quarterly Publication of the National Association of Social Workers,* 3:10–14.

Rosengarten L (1980). Case management: A definition in historical perspective. *Issues in Service Coordination for the Elderly with Developmental Disabilities:* 8–21.

Rubenstein S, Wilson M (1982). Collaboration in a hospital: The case of the dying woman. *Journal of Gerontological Social Work,* 5:169–179. Also in G Getzel (Ed.) *Gerontological Social Work—Long Term Care.* New York:Haworth Press (1982).

Schwartz P (1983). On support groups. *The National Neurofibromatosis Foundation, Inc.,* 6:1,3.

Schwartz P (1987). Central nervous system form neurofibromatosis. In K Post, J Jaffee, P Reubens, AH Kutscher, I Hoffmeister, K Muraszka, LF Post (Eds.). *Acute, Chronic and Terminal Care in Neurosurgery.* Springfield, IL: CC Thomas:109–114.

Shapiro V, Gisynski M (1989). Ghosts in the nursery revisited. *Child and Adolescent Social Work,* 6(1):18–37.

Shein L (1987). *Social Workers' Perception and Practices in Relation to the Children of Psychiatrically Hospitalized Patients.* Dissertation. New York University.

Siegel ME (1984). A child, death and sesame street. *Social Work Oncology Network New York Bulletin IV,* Spring/Summer.

Siegel ME, Koplin H (1984). *More Than a Friend: Dogs with a Purpose*. New York: Walker and Co.

Siegel ME (1984). Children's reaction to death of grandparents. *Archives of the Foundation of Thanatology, 10*.

Siegel ME (1985). To tell the truth. *Archives of the Foundation of Thanatology, 11*.

Siegel ME (1986). Suffering: Psychological and Social Aspects in Loss Grief and Care. In R Debillis, E Marcus, A Kutscher, C Torres, V Barrett, ME Siegel (Eds.). New York: Haworth Press.

Siegel ME (1986). What shall we tell the children. *Archives of the Foundation of Thanatology, 12*.

Siegel ME (1987). After the last goodbye. *Archives of the Foundation of Thanatology:13*.

Siegel ME (1987). Their sorrow, our sorrow. In R Debillis, GR Hyman, I Seeland, A Kutscher, A Kemberg, ME Siegel, L Kutscher (Eds.). *Psychosocial Aspects of Chemotherapy in Cancer Care*. New York: Haworth Press.

Siegel ME (1987). The patient, family and staff. In R Debellis, GR Hyman, I Seeland, A Kutscher, A Kemberg, ME Siegel, L Kutscher (Eds.). *Psychosocial Aspects of Chemotherapy in Cancer Care*. New York: Haworth Press.

Siegel ME (1987). Scared, puzzled, and angry even when I'm not sad. *Archives of the Foundation of Thanatology, 13*.

Siegel ME (1988). *Psychiatric Aspects of Terminal Illness*. Philadelphia, PA: Charles Press.

Siegel ME (1988). Goodbye Kitty. In WJ Kay (Ed.). *Euthanasia of the Companion Animal*. Philadelphia, PA: Charles Press.

Siegel ME (1988). Children's reactions to deaths of grandparents and great grandparents: Case histories. In O Margolis, A Kutscher, E Marcus, HC Raether, VR Pine, I Seeland, D Cherico (Eds.). *Grief and the Loss of Adult Child*. New York: Praeger.

Silberman J, Kornfield P, Landman L, Stern D, Gross H, Genkins G (Eds.) (1983). Psychosocial aspects of myasthenia gravis. In *Psychosocial Aspects of Muscular Dystrophy and Allied Diseases*. Springfield, IL:177–182.

Silberman JM (1986). *Spouses' Perception of the Impact of Myasthenia Gravis on Marital Interaction*. Dissertation. New York University.

Silverton M (1988). *Assessing mental health problems in minority boys*. Dissertation. Dissertation Abstract International:48.

Steidl J, Mandelbaum E (1987). Case studies and economics: Integrating a family-systems approach in adult medical settings. *Family Systems Medicine, 5*:238–245.

Walther V (1989). Post-partum depression: An overview. *NASW Forum, 9*:1–7.

Weissman A (1986). Linkage in direct practice. *Encyclopedia of Social Work*. Silver Springs, MD: National Association of Social Workers, 2:47–50.

Weissman A (1989). A social worker comments: Quality referrals. *Social Work in Health Care, 13*:51–56.

Young AT (1980). Social Work Services. In LM Aledort, JP Maher, JM Cohen, NW Lyman (Eds.). *Outpatient Medicine*. New York: Raven Press:12–16.

Young AT (1985). Commentary on 'knowledge and skill requirements for social work practice in maternal and child health.' In K Kumane (Ed.). *Proceedings: Public Health Social Work in Maternal and Child Health: A Forward Plan*. June.

Zofnass J (1982). *Social Workers' Attitudes and Behavioral Intentions Toward the Elderly*. Dissertation. Adelphi University School of Social Work.

1990s

Aledort L, Weiss H, Parker CT, Levi J, Simon R (1990). The life-style interventions in the young. In S Shumaker, *et al.* (Eds.). *The Handbook of Health Behavior Change.* New York: Springer:293–314.

Berrier J, Sperling R, Preisinger J, Mason J, Walther V (1991). HIV/AIDS education in a prenatal clinic: An assessment. *AIDS Education and Prevention,* 3:100–117.

Black RB (1991). Women's voices after pregnancy loss: Couples' patterns of communication and support. *Social Work in Health Care, 16*:19–36.

Black RB (1991). Social work practice with children and adolescents with chronic illness and disabilities. In S Bardfield, RB Black (Eds.). *Social Work Practice with Maternal and Child Health: Populations at Risk, a Casebook.* New York: Columbia University School of Social Work:165–173.

Black RB, Weiss JA (1990). Genetic support groups and social workers as partners. *Health and Social Work, 15*:91–99.

Black RB, Weiss JA (1991). Chronic physical illness and disability. In A Gitterman (Ed.). *Handbook of Social Work Practice with Vulnerable Populations, 4*:137–164.

Blumenfield S, Simon EP, Bennett C (1991). The legal clinic: Helping social workers master the legal environment in health care. *Social Work in Health Care, 16*(2).

Cipriano LA (1991). Psychoanalytic perspectives on substance abuse: Implications for treatment program planning and social policy. *Social Work in Health Care, 15*(3).

Cuzzi L (1991). Management of the borderline substance abuser. In E Lowenkopf, S Klebanow (Eds.). *Money and Mind.* New York: Plenum:197–205.

Davidson KW, Clarke S (Eds.) (1990). *Social Work in Health Care: A Handbook for Practice.* New York: Haworth Press.

Dobrof J, Umpierre M, Rocha L, Silverton M (1990). Group work in a primary care medical setting. *Health and Social Work, 15*(1):32–37.

Dobrof J (1991). DRGs and the social worker's role in discharge planning. *Social Work in Health Care, 16*(2):37–54.

Eskin V, Zilberfein F (1991). Treating the hospitalized medically ill holocaust survivor. *New York Metro Chapter Forum* 2:10–11.

Fisher B (1991). Coping with a child's chronic illness: Mr. and Mrs. Hoto. *Social Work Practice with Maternal and Child Health: Populations at Risk, A Casebook.* New York: Columbia University School of Social Work:185–190.

Gantt A, Levine J (1990). The roles of social work in psycho-biological research. *Social Work in Health Care, 15*:63–75.

Garwood L (1991). A child with AIDS: Eddy Fuentes. In S Bardfield, RB Black (Eds.). *Social Work Practice with Maternal and Child Health: Populations at Risk, A Casebook.* New York: Columbia University School of Social Work:85–100.

Greenfield D, Walther V (1991). Psychological aspects of recurrent pregnancy loss. *Infertility and Reproductive Medicine Clinics of North America,* 2:235–247.

Holden G, Moncher MS, Schinke SP, Barker KC (1990). Self-efficacy of children, and adolescents: A meta-analysis. *Psychological Reports, 66*:1044–1046.

Holden G, Moncher MS. (1990). Substance abuse. In AS Bellack, E Kazdin, H Hersen (Eds.). *International Handbook of Behavior Modification and Therapy.* New York: Plenum Press:869–880.

Inniss P (1991). Pulmonary therapy and rehabilitation. In F Haas, K Axin. *Principles and Practice.* Baltimore, MD, 16:289–300.

Jacobs E (1991). An adolescent mother: Molly. *Social Work Practice with Maternal and Child Health: Populations at Risk, A Casebook.* New York: Columbia University School of Social Work:37–47.

Laureano M, Poliandro E (1991). Understanding cultural values of Latino male alcoholics and their families: A culture sensitive model. *Chemical Dependency: Theoretical Approaches and Strategies.* New York: Haworth Press:4:137–155.

Mailick MD (1991). Re-assessing assessment in clinical social work practice. *Smith College Studies in Social Work,* 62:4–19.

Mailick M (1990). Social work practice with adolescents: Theoretical saturation. In H Weissman (Ed.). *Creativity and Innovation in Social Work.* Silver Springs, MD: National Association of Social Workers.

Mason J (1991). High risk pregnancy: Kathie O'Hara. In S Bardfield, RB Black (Eds.). *Social Work Practice with Maternal and Child Health: Populations at Risk, A Casebook.* New York: Columbia University School of Social Work:49–55.

Mason J, Preisinger J, Sperling R, Walther V, Berrier J, Evans V (1991). Incorporating HIV education and counseling into routine prenatal care. *AIDS Education and Prevention,* 3:118–123.

Moncher MS, Holden G, Schinke SP, J Palleja (1990). Behavioral family treatment of the substance abusing Hispanic adolescent. In EI Fiendler, GR Kalfus (Eds.). *Adolescent Behavior Therapy Handbook.* New York: Springer, 13:329–349.

Moncher MS, Holden G, Schinke SP (1991). Tobacco addiction: Correlates, prevention and treatment. In E Freedman (Ed.). *The Addiction Process: Effective Social Work Approaches.*

Moncher MS, Holden G, Schinke SP (1991). Psychosocial correlates of adolescent substance abuse: A review of current etiological constructs. *International Journal of the Addictions,* 26:377–414.

Moncher MS, Holden G, Trimble JE (1990). Substance abuse among native American youth. *Journal of Consulting and Clinical Psychology,* 58(4):415–418.

Nathan A, Razin A (1991). Suicidal behavior among inner-city Hispanic adolescent females. *General Hospital Psychiatry,*13:45–58.

O'Dowd MA, Zofnass J (1991). Neuropsychiatric and psychosocial factors in the rehabilitation of patients with AIDs. In J Mukand (Ed.). *Rehabilitation for Patients with HIV Disease.* New York: McGraw Hill, Inc.:199–215.

Preminger MD, Gordon ML (1991). Support and psycho-education for parents of hospitalized mentally ill children. *Health and Social Work,* 16(1):11–17.

Rosenberg G (1991). Editorial: The known and unknown about the chronically ill. *Social Work in Health Care,* 15(5):1–3.

Siegel ME (1990). What about me?: Unrecognized loss and sanctioned grief: The nature and counseling of unacknowledged loss. In V Pine, O Margolis, K Doka, A Kutcher, D Schaefer, ME Siegel, D Cherico (Eds). *Archives of the Foundation of Thanatology.* Springfield, IL: CC Thomas.

Stein E, Wade K, Smith D (1991). Clinical support groups that work. *Journal of the Association of Nurses in AIDS Care (Janac),* 2:29–36.

Strugger M (1991). An overwhelmed mother neglects her son: Susan. In S Bardfield, RB Black (Eds.). *Social Work Practice with Maternal and Child Health: Populations at Risk, A Casebook.* New York: Columbia University School of Social Work:263–274.

Walther V (1991). Emerging roles of social work in perinatal services. *Social Work in Health Care,* 15(2):35–48.

Weiss HM, Simon R, Levi J, *et al.* (1991). Compliance in a comprehensive hemophilia center and its implication for home care. *Family Systems Medicine, 9*:112–120.

Woodrow R (1991). Social work practice with families with AIDS: Population at risk. In S Bardfield, RB Black (Eds.). *Social Work Practice with Maternal and Child Health: Populations at Risk, A Casebook.* New York: Columbia University School of Social Work:59–71.

ETHICS

1970s

Bosch S, Rehr H, Lewis H (1978). Some suggested remedies, resolutions and further deliberations. In H Rehr (Ed.). *Ethical Dilemmas in Health Care: A Professional Search for Solutions.* New York: Prodist:79–85.

Dana B (1978). Value dilemmas in the delivery of social heath services: Caring, coping and curing. In H Rehr (Ed.). *Ethical Dilemmas in Health Care: A Professional Search for Solutions.* New York: Prodist:25–32.

Horowitz G, Maher J (1978). Values and ethical dilemmas in relation to the delivery of social health care to the aging. In H Rehr (Ed.). *Ethical Dilemmas in Health Care: A Professional Search for Solutions.* New York: Prodist:63–75.

Maglin A (1978). Social values and psychotherapy. *Catalyst, 3.*

Rehr H (Ed.) (1978). *Ethical Dilemmas in Health Care: A Professional Search for Solutions.* New York: Prodist.

Rehr H, Bosch S (1978). A professional search into values and ethics in health care delivery. In H Rehr (Ed.). *Ethical Dilemmas in Health Care: A Professional Search for Solutions.* New York: Prodist:35–62.

Shulman L, Rosenberg G (1976). Political skill in social work practice. In A Lurie, G Rosenberg (Eds.). *Social Work in Mental Health.* New Hyde Park, NY: L.I. Jewish-Hillside Medical Center, *XI*:97–110.

1980s

Blumenfield S, Lowe JI (1987). Data, values and decision-making: A template for analyzing ethical dilemmas in discharge planning. *Health and Social Work, 12*:47–56.

Dana B (1980). Social development for social justice: The health-justice connection. *St. Louis University School of Social Service—Proceedings of 50th Anniversary Lecture Series Theme: Social Development for Social Justice.*

Ravich R (1986). Patient advocacy. In J Marks (Ed.). *Advocacy in Health Care.* Clifton, NJ: Humana Press:51–60.

Rehr H (1981). Ethical dilemmas in health care delivery. *Journal of Social Work Process, 14*:55–63.

Riecken HW, Ravich R (1982). Informed consent to biomedical research in veterans administration. *Journal of the American Medical Association, 248*(3):344–348.

Young AT (1987). Discharge planning and ethical dilemmas. *Discharge Planning Update, 7*: 3–4.

Young AT (1987). A delicate balance: Teenage and parent rights and responsibilities. *Proceedings on Adolescent Issues: Pregnancy, Parenting, Health, Maternal and Child Health Division.* USDHEW:11–14.

Zofnass J (1982). *Social Workers' Attitudes and Behavioral Intentions Toward the Elderly.* Dissertation. Adelphi University School of Social Work.

1990s

Bernstein SR (1991). *Managing Contracted Services in the Non-Profit Agency: Administrative Ethical and Political Issues.* Philadelphia, PA: Temple University Press.

Blumenfield S, Simon EP, Bennett C (1991). The legal clinic: Helping social workers master the legal environment in health care. *Social Work in Health Care,* 16(2):7–9.

Laureano M, Poliandro E (1991). Understanding cultural values of Latino male alcoholics and their families: A culture sensitive model. *Chemical Dependency: Theoretical Approaches and Strategies.* New York: Haworth Press, 4:137–155.

Lowe J (1991). *Letting the People Decide: A Study of the Citizens' Committee on Biomedical Ethics, Inc. and Its Citizen-leaders (Citizens' Committee on Biomedical Ethics Inc.).* Dissertation. Rutgers, The State University of New Jersey.

Ravich R (1990). Patients' rights in breast surgery. In A Gross, D Soto (Eds.). *Women Talk About Surgery,* New York: Potter:300–307.

Ravich R (1990). Patients' rights in gynecological surgery. In A Gross, D Soto (Eds.). *Women Talk About Their Surgery.* New York: Potter:308–317.

Siegel ME (1990). Rites of Passage/Rights of Passage. In A Kutscher, S Bess, S Klagsbrun, ME Siegel, DJ Cherico, L Kutscher, D Peretz, FE Selder (Eds.). *For the Bereaved: The Road to Recovery.* Philadelphia, PA: Charles Press.

4

Program Development, Organization, and Administrative Directions

Gary Rosenberg, Susan Blumenfield, and Helen Rehr

"To function effectively in an environment increasingly driven by the economics of 'managed competition,' social work directors must thoroughly understand the contents and contributions of our profession, maintain a sensitivity to professional ethics and individual consumer health care rights, and exercise competent business judgment" (Spitzer, 1995; p. 106).

Rosenberg and Weissman (1995) forecast the implications for social work in a changing health care system. They note the drastic reorganization occurring in the industry as it emulates changes in corporate America. Employers and insurers are creating new health care systems for lower costs. The federal government failed to achieve health care reform, and freedom of choice has shifted to a payment choice system. But Rosenberg and Weissman are not necessarily negative about the future of health care. They see a health care system:

- that is vertically integrated, including programs that deal with prevention, wellness, and health education, and acute and long term care;
- that will be regionally based and serve wide geographic areas, in a linked network of social-health care organizations;
- in which capitation and controlled managed-care reimbursement will be the primary payment plans; and
- in which changes are expected to cut or to control rises in costs.

As they see it, this new health care system involves a shift from inpatient acute care to ambulatory services. Today's major emphasis on tertiary specialized care will shift to a major delivery system of primary care; the number of specialists will be reduced; and early diagnosis and treatment and prevention services will be emphasized (pp. 111–116).

This new health care system is fast upon us. Institutions are downsizing, streamlining, and changing the way work is done. They are identifying the unnecessary and eliminating duplication. Financial considerations are driving operations, and higher (and varied) levels of productivity are expected. Health care systems are expanding into networks of organizations; administration will flatten in some characteristics, but expand in new organizational designs. As institutions regain control of their financial base, the hope is that they will turn to considerations of access and quality. They will form coalitions with health care providers, business, and consumers to work with commercially based payers to secure professional standards and sound, comprehensive services.

Professional groups face uncertainty about their continuing roles in this new health care environment. They are expected to justify their services. Institutions are cross-training staffs with the expectation that multipurpose personnel will reduce costs, reduce the size of professional groups, and eliminate professional boundaries. Turf conflicts are resurfacing. Professionals will need to redefine themselves, and professional boundaries will need to be clarified.

THE CHALLENGE

To be effective in a health care organization, a social work administrator has responsibilities that necessarily extend beyond skillful management of the social work department. Social work administrators, particularly those who demonstrate quality leadership and administrative competency, must assume responsibilities for a wide range of services in health care settings. Among these are managing volunteers, patient representatives, crisis intervention, employee assistance, wellness, rehabilitation, community outreach, health education programs, training and support groups for staff, and even hospital administrative functions. Clinical skill is essential to understand the dynamics of interaction with others; it transfers readily to administrative savvy.

A social work department must develop a clear-cut relationship between the institution's mission and its services and tasks. The primary mission of social work in health settings is to contribute to quality patient care outcomes. To this end, essential administrative goals are to build professional self-confidence, maintain social work values and integrity, and serve as an advocate for patients. Knowing one's staff, its level of performance, and the institutional system is critical. To know patient needs, the community, and available resources to meet those needs also is essential. Collaboration with other department leaders contributes to development of effective services. A good leader knows how to negotiate and establish administrative credibility by demonstrating fiscal responsibility and by identifying the issues requiring advocacy or change on patients' behalf. Staff must demonstrate that they can produce quality services and achieve sound patient outcomes despite shrinking resources (Bixby, 1995; pp. 3–20). Staff must therefore be stakeholders in the institution's mission and have or develop problem-solving skills that are supported by knowledge, self-confidence, professional identity, and solid leadership.

In contributing to the scope, direction, and planning of services, social work leaders must:

- know what information to gather, how to gather it, and how to use it selectively;
- be professionally accountable, using evaluation measurements;
- have communication and negotiating skills and the capacity to collaborate with other health care professionals and administrators;
- be able to recognize (and reach) short- and long-term goals;
- initiate patient-care programs such as consumer advocacy and employee assistance programs;
- be able to make decisions quickly, with self-confidence;
- have monitoring and organizing skills;
- prepare staff for self-directed practice;
- have financial awareness, business acumen, and the skills to function effectively despite shrinking resources;
- have strategic planning and marketing skills that make social work services visible and that create awareness among the institution's professional and lay communities;
- identify with the population they serve, particularly the needy, and relate to organizational needs and priorities; and
- be able to manage their time and the use of self.

Blumenfeld (1995) notes that an administrative–staff partnership is required to "balance the demands of staff for professional integrity with the demands of the hospital and regulatory bodies for cost containment and length-of-stay controls, balancing fiscal realities with needs for resource" (p. 25) for patients and for quality staff performance. A department needs to be goal-focused. Visible leadership that promotes social services is essential. Ongoing enhancement of clinical skills is required to achieve quality performance and program development. Departmental practice and programs must be reviewed continuously. An administrator needs to find the tools to identify vulnerable areas of patient need. Practice studies that generate data about services can advance quality performance and help evaluate programs for cost effectiveness.

A focus on populations as well as on individuals is a helpful perspective. Screening for high risk and drawing on other public health studies can provide an administrator with a programmatic emphasis. Such information coupled with financial know-how can lead to developing programs for vulnerable groups in need. Administrators cannot function in a unilinear direction; that is, from the top down. They engage a staff to serve patients, and it is staff in partnership with administration that reviews practice. Good leaders use power to influence, and they sort and use information selectively. Speed in decision making is necessary, requiring information and self-confidence. Simplicity in communication and in conceptualization improves the planning and design implementation process. Offering staff the voice to assess their own performance and to recommend changes helps them in turn to implement change. Leaders need to find the way "to create a fit between aspirations and resources" (Blumenfield, 1995; p. 35).

Hospital-based social work essentially is a matrix organization, operating with dual responsibilities to the service unit and to social work administration (Mayer 1995; p. 70). Social workers are professionally accountable to the department and to the unit of service. The debate regarding the effectiveness of a "unified" versus a "unitized" structure for social work services (Siegel & Knee, 1959) is revisited today as institutions downsize and restructure service delivery systems and develop patient-centered care units staffed by personnel who are trained cross-functionally. The concept of a decentralized unit operation, borrowed from corporate America, is based on the premise that people closest to the product line can make the most cost-effective recommendations. But sick persons in a patient care unit are not commodities in a fixed production line. They are unique individuals with unique needs.

Today almost all health care providers have articulated the need to be responsive to patients' biopsychosocial needs. Social work has been successful in bringing this perspective to institutional providers. But social work administrators must sharpen their knowledge to identify vulnerable persons, secure their access to relevant care, and help them further their heath status by engaging in self-care. At the same time, social work administrators must collaborate with their health care colleagues to ensure more comprehensive programs of care for patients and families.

A knowledge of complex organizations and social systems is imperative. Social work administrators must correlate the needs of the department's clientele with the institution's actual and prospective population. Because institutional expectations and client needs sometimes conflict (particularly when those needs exceed or are outside the boundaries of reimbursement), social work administrators must have broad knowledge of external resources, and social workers must thoroughly assess the family–patient relationship to reconcile differences.

A complex organization is comprised of multiple constituencies. Social workers interact with numerous professions and lay groups, including doctors, nurses, administrators, board members, financial officers, paraprofessionals, support staff, and patients and their families. Knowing all the different groups and their philosophies and expectations is critical to effective communication and collaboration. Social workers also interact with numerous external groups, such as regulators, payers, community agents, and so forth. To relate effectively, social work administrators must shift from a process focus, which slows decision making, to a planning and resolution focus.

Despite the numerous changes occurring in health care today and anticipated in the future, a centralized department of social work (or of nursing, pharmacy, rehabilitation, or physical or occupational therapy) should prevail to support the professional functions that best serve people. Social workers assigned to units of patient care are team members with dual accountability: to the patient-care program and its leadership and to the profession through a centralized social work system. Centralization permits a unified approach to emerging patient care needs, maintaining standards, accountability and quality improvement, the ongoing education of professionals, assessment of programs, the rise of multiple constituencies, and community and health care system needs. Social work, when unified, can be in the community helping to identify the vulnerable through risk screening, by community outreach, by seeking ways to help those in the community use services appropriately, and by implementing programs of health education and maintenance.

ONE DEPARTMENT'S GROWTH AND DEVELOPMENT

At the end of 1953, as it broadened its concept of medical care, Mount Sinai responded to the recommendation of the auxiliary board to develop a professional social work department. Over a period of more than 40 years, the department developed and grew, modifying its mission and goals in concert with changes occurring in the environment as well as within the institution. Today, in the latter half of the 1990s, the department is completely professionalized. It provides services to hospitalized patients as well as those in ambulatory programs and in the community, answers to hospital administration, has a seat on the medical and community boards, and continues a collaborative relationship with the auxiliary board. It participates actively in education and research and has earned a national and international reputation for service.

When the medical school was established in 1966, the division of social work in the department of community medicine was created and a number of staff received faculty appointments. In 1968, the division was honored with the creation of an endowed chair and a Professorship in Community Medicine (Social Work), a first. The endowed chair in social work to this day is the only one that exists in a medical school.

The department currently is staffed by 175 social workers and a support staff of 25. Of the department's professional social workers, 61 have been reviewed over time by the appointments and promotions committee and appointed to faculty status in the medical school on the basis of credentials and expectations comparable to those for medical staff appointees.

Throughout its history, social work administrators and their collegial staff focused on five areas, demonstrated in the writings collected in this inventory:

- enhancing the department's services by developing new social work services and new programs;
- examining administrative practices and the contribution of the clinical enterprise and seeking cost-effective social work services;
- bringing a social-health component to the hospital's delivery of services; in developing consultative and collaborative relationships;
- responding to consumers, by creating a lay-professional partnership through enhanced networking with the hospital's community and with the many social and health organizations committed to social-health care enhancement; and
- establishing key roles in social work education, medical education, and research, by assuming teaching responsibilities and curriculum development.

THE RELEVANT LITERATURE

ENHANCING SERVICES

In the late 1950s and 1960s, social work provided an important contribution to broadening the concept of medical care through introduction of social-health programs. These programs were developed with the realization that all medical care requires a biopsychosocial-environmental dimension in diagnosis and that social diagnosis must be supportive to ensure comprehensive treatment. A psychosocial orientation to care also was deemed essential to enhance motivation if patients were to achieve optimal outcomes. A seminal article written in the early 1950s attested to the "necessity" of social work services in a hospital, shifting the emphasis from a biomedical model of care to a biopsychosocial model. By the mid-1960s, the hospital supported the new philosophy through the increasing development of multidisciplinary programs.

What occurred in each of four decades that prompted social workers to design and contribute to programs that affect social-health care? Whether by study of, observation of, or experience with patients and families, social workers—with other health care practitioners—witness the impact of illness and disability on individuals and families. They see the need to work with patients and families to help them achieve a quality of life that accommodates for physical and social functioning limitations.

Social workers analyze problem situations in terms of client needs, institutional deterrents to services, provider-client interrelationships, or community gaps in the provision of services. As a result of simple, applied studies and reflection, social workers have been able to translate their observations into a systematic response that leads to change in program, to new programs, or to enhanced partnerships between clients and providers. This pattern of reflective study predated continuous quality improvement assessments. Many programs that social workers initiated are in collaboration with other health care providers (and the institution) and with community agencies.

NEW SERVICES

Team collaboration and consultation were implemented as basic social work functions in the late 1950s and early 1960s. In partnership with local schools of social work, field curricula were expanded and students were involved in a growing number of social work programs. Studies to enhance practice and programs were supported. In an early study, social workers observed that hospital services were fragmented and patients faced obstacles in getting care. As a result, a new concept was pioneered: the patient representative program, which smooths the flow of services and improves communication between providers and patients. Patient representative services have flourished in other institutions, but are not without critics, particularly among social workers in hospital settings who see similarities between the patient representative program and social work services and who fear the program could preempt part of social work's domain.

Social work administrative studies produced information that people in its communities were not getting the medical care they needed. In the early 1960s, the federal Model Cities program was developed in the local community. Social work administration helped the institution create a community board, served by a majority of hospital consumers, to explore appropriate programs with providers. The community board still exists and enjoys the active participation of community residents who also use the institution's services.

In conjunction with colleagues in community medicine, social workers participated in local school health planning, in networking to improve access to health care for Medicaid-eligible families, and in developing community health planning with community members. The pattern of working with the community to determine needs and implement programs advanced over time. The social-health advocacy program was developed in the late 1960s following the Pearl and Reissman (1965) recognition of community persons as best able to serve their neighbors, and continues today. In the 1980s, social work initiated a community relations health department, which was institutionalized within the hospital to expand its roles with community agencies and make the institution's services relevant to community needs.

NEW PROGRAMS

Social work demonstrated a need to institute new programs as early as the 1950s. For example, social work administration recognized that long-term dependency in illness was a common occurrence addressed poorly by social workers in health settings and those in community agencies. Social work developed a social-health treatment approach for chronic illness with major emphasis on reality problems and on enhancing the individual's level of social functioning. Although physical limitations were seen as critical, social-environmental needs also were recognized and addressed. Social functioning was identified as the fundamental factor in achieving a better quality-of-life. The polio epidemic crystallized these concerns and the social-health focus on care prompted development of the doctor-nurse-social worker team in a multidisciplinary center to serve victims and their families. Social workers began to leave the hospital base and go out into the community. A program of comprehensive care for chronically ill patients and their families was initiated and followed patients to their homes. Guidelines developed 30 years ago to serve discharged patients and their families have been modified as new information, market conditions, and resources emerged.

The same requirement for a continuum of comprehensive service that surfaced for chronic disability developed for newborns with brain defects. Orientation of professional staff promoted a holistic perception of patients' needs and appropriate services. A joint hospital-social work-family agency effort supported the conviction that care must follow patients and families. Adding homemaker services to hospital social work service delivery supported the 'at home' program for patients.

Recognizing that patients need their families to support their posthospital care, social work initiated family counseling. This family-focused care led to introduction of family therapy on behalf of patients with hemophilia, speech disorders, cancer, and other disorders and diseases.

In the 1960s social work leadership recognized the need for utilization studies to determine patterns in the use of institutional and social services. Understanding these patterns could enhance practice and the need for new programs. For example, a series of studies of unwed mothers recognized the need for health education and health services for different subgroups of this population and led to new programs. The lack of community services for black teenagers, and black young women multiparas, compared to the opportunity and choice available to white women, meant that these women were seriously disadvantaged. Black women were expected to take their newborns into their mothers' homes, while white women could elect for adoption or other choices. Prevention and health education came to be seen as public health needs, and avoiding additional pregnancies became a component in a health education program for teenage primiparas.

Providers deemed chronic multiple clinic users who presented themselves with multiple complaints as a "hard core" group. The hospital administration and the board of trustees, based on the recommendation of a physician and a social worker, underwrote a comprehensive care program that involved a multidisciplinary team comprised of a doctor, a nurse, and a social worker. The program was terminated after two and a half years because it was not received well by physicians, who thought it competed with their private practices. In addition, the program's staff found itself ill-prepared to deal with multiple patient demands, and complained of burnout.

A group counseling program was developed for the frail elderly, and a study of outcomes of group therapy revealed strengthening in their self-containment. This early program was the foundation of the social work emphasis on group services that are both age- and illness-related. A therapeutic community for mentally ill patients in which an opportunity for self-government was offered proved successful. Self-governing units marked the beginning of milieu therapy in psychiatry. A study of abortion seekers led to development of a pregnancy assessment clinic to identify the psychological risk to these women and offer counseling to assist in decision making and in prevention of unwanted pregnancies.

The social work department created a home care support program for frail elderly, encouraged a coordinated continuum of care for discharged, sick aging patients, and developed a case-management approach to care via a geriatric team that continues to serve the population and enhance hospital staff's knowledge in its work with the elderly. Consultation, education, and a private geriatric social work service are based in the institution and made available to health care professionals, their inpatients, and patients seen in their private offices. Social workers adopted coordination of services as a function to eliminate fragmentation and help patients navigate the maze of an increasingly complex institutional environment. Elder volunteers were brought in to serve the sick elderly. Developing oral histories is used in an affiliated nursing home as a life-review therapy. A foster grandparents program for children and adolescents in an acute psychiatric service was introduced successfully.

A new hand-carried form for discharged patients to help them receive ongoing care when they enter a clinic forecasts diagnoses and ongoing needs. When patient representatives demonstrated a need to help deaf patients and staff communicate with each other, a pictograph was introduced. An innovative preadmission screening process involves patients in a group session to determine the need for inpatient admission to psychiatry. The process demonstrated that patients can be supported while waiting for admission.

The Impact of Employee Strikes

In the late 1950s, labor-management problems resulted in labor strikes against hospitals. In working with hospitalized patients during the crisis, social workers developed a new function—triaging those inpatients who could leave the hospital without detriment to their health, working with patients and families to reduce anxiety exacerbated by the strike, and in direct floor care such as meal delivery, feeding assistance, running elevators, and working the back of the hospital to ensure continuity of medical care. Almost 30 years later, in again examining the effects of an employee strike on patient care, a study found that housekeeping and dietary services were most affected, while medical, nursing, and social work were least affected. It appears that professionals are motivated to ensure that the care of the sick continues during a strike. The introduction of triaging of inpatients for early discharge with adequate home support was successful in reducing the impact of the strike on services. It also fostered development of social work roles in other crisis situations.

CENTRALIZED VERSUS DECENTRALIZED SERVICES

The issue of a unified versus a unitized department was prevalent in the field of medical social work from its beginnings. Not only were medical and psychiatric social work services separated in the same institution, but many social work services in hospitals in the country answered to a unit manager, most often a medical chief. The institution supported the value of a unified social work department and recognized that professionalization, quality of care, sound distribution of services, accountability, and continuing staff education and development could best be maintained in a centralized department. The benefits of a unified department have been demonstrated over the years. However, the recent, dramatic restructuring of hospitals has caused the issue of centralization to resurface, albeit in a somewhat different context. Autonomous unit teams are being introduced with medical, nursing, social work, or business leadership. Social workers in the new patient-centered care units may be assigned to one or two units, responsible to unit leaders. It appears that serious attempts are being made to preserve some of the benefits of centralization, and unity plus centralized accountability are projected for the majority of nonmedical professionals.

CASEFINDING

Delays and gaps in services were discovered in pioneering studies of referral of patients and families to social services. The introduction of casefinding, a public health modality of drawing on high social-risk screening techniques, guaranteed timely access to care. Social-risk screening became a clinical indicator of quality-of-care, supported and surveyed by the Joint Commission on Accreditation of Healthcare Organizations. Social work assumed social-risk screening as a major function in its casefinding process. It provided its own casefinding in conjunction with a referral system. A serendipitous outcome was the enhancement of social work studies as social work assumed professional responsibility for finding those at-risk.

EVALUATION OF QUALITY AND COST

Administrators must have a keen commitment to the quality and cost-effectiveness of care. They must routinely examine the cost of social services delivery, drawing on financial management and cost-benefit concepts.

Costing services and analyses of patients at-risk have led to different patterns of service allocation and to the recognition that certain groups in need of health care services were not receiving them. The department learned budgetary practices and revenue sources, and established a management information system to review revenue and expense patterns for inpatients and ambulatory care.

Although early work devised staffing standards according to bed capacity, pre- and at-admission high social-risk screening were later developed and encouraged awareness of "severity of illness" as a variable for access to social work services. Through high social-risk screening social workers took responsibility for casefinding, which led to greater visibility of social work services to all constituencies.

MARKETING

Marketing social work services helped publicize the social-health concept of care and provide services irrespective of patient income status. The department was able to generate revenue and create additional income-producing social work positions that allowed expansion of social work services within the medical center. Development of an internal medicine hospital group practice led to an expanded role for social work in the fee-for-service program.

PRIMARY CARE GROUP PRACTICE

Most recently, social work's roles have been redefined in a primary care group practice based on a program that failed 20 years earlier. The original program attempted to serve multiple clinic users with multiple complaints in a coordinated service. Today the group serves a case mix of sick and less sick patients and prepares and trains health care professionals to offer coordinated quality care. The program is placed in its own location outside hospital doors and has resulted in reorganization of ambulatory clinics in general and integration of the group practice with social work, which has demonstrated successful outcomes for patients and the service.

In the future social work will assume responsibility for care of groups of chronically ill patients, who have moved from inpatient to ambulatory care and require psychosocial intervention. In moving outside the traditional hospital setting, social work now emphasizes the promotion of health education and prevention. It works to empower and strengthen the geographic community as well as government and community relations, organizational effectiveness, and corporate health programs such as wellness, fitness, and employee assistance.

DISCHARGE PLANNING

Programs to enhance the quality and character of discharge planning for patients have been undertaken: an interim home care program demonstrated reduced length-of-stay while providing at-home supports. Recent articles describe work with HIV and AIDS patients and benefits of support groups for nurses who work with these patients. Serving the elderly and disabled through a trained therapeutic companion program has been successful. The benefits of a coalition between patients and social workers to address patients with genetic disorders illustrates another professional-client partnership. Perinatal social work as a new field of practice is described in conjunction with newly developed technology and biomedical treatment. Perinatal preventive services were introduced into the hospital's local community as social workers work with high-risk mothers-to-be. As primary care doctors and specialists introduce health education and maintenance in their practice a special content knowledge for social work services is demonstrated.

CONSUMER SATISFACTION

The patient and/or family are the key actors in the relationship with a social worker. In its work in quality assurance and quality improvement, the department developed instruments to evaluate its services through consumer satisfaction surveys and provider opinions. Consumer and family member reactions led to management staff review and enhanced programs in social services and in the institution at large. The correlation of consumer with provider opinion of care led to better social work practice. The medical center recognized the design, development, and implementation of a social work services' patient satisfaction survey as an important innovation and established a survey center as a separate department under the leadership of a research-trained social worker. The department is responsible for undertaking all hospitalwide surveys of patients, staff, medical students, and physicians.

CONCLUSION

Social-health programs are an integral component of social work in medical institutions. Their development and integration into institutional programs attest to social work's contribution to the hospital's services.

Social work administrators contributed to the enhancement of institutional programs, to institutional socialization, and to indirect cost savings and revenue production. Opportunities to move into various roles in hospital administration resulted. The assessment of institutional problems made social work administration aware that it had been defining itself too narrowly and distancing itself from a comprehensive approach to patient health care needs. The institution recognized that competency in the management of social services and the growth in social-health programs developed by social workers enhanced patient care and cost-effectiveness. The institution also recognized its need to be socialized and to ensure greater individualized patient care. Social work skills were deemed essential, and social work's leaders were drawn into hospital administration.

The focus was not limited to enhancing patient well-being, but included improving the management-employee relationship as well as training to achieve new objectives. As social work administrators became more involved in hospital administration roles, they sought additional skills to reinforce their capabilities to address new and expanded functions. They focused on development of services and on social-health programs, enhancement of clinical skills and cost-effective practice, socialization of the institution and its providers, social work's autonomy and its response to consumers and the community, and key roles in medical education and research.

From its very beginnings, the social work profession has been motivated by patient needs. The social work product—skills in mediating systems, in advocating for entitlements, and in assessing the biopsychosocial needs of patients and families in primary, secondary, and tertiary care—is continually strengthened to be relevant to patients, to the community, and to the institution. Emphases and staffing patterns might change, and other structural arrangements might be necessary, but the basic product reflects patient needs. For social work's relevance to be understood, for its boundaries to remain intact, hospital management must recognize that social work is flexible, creative, and collaborative. Social work administration must make new alliances, communicate in a thoughtful and supportive manner, reassure social work staff that their professional integrity is intact, and be ready for change in assignments and practice emphases, but not in philosophy, values, and ethics (Blumenfield, 1995; pp. 35–36).

MOUNT SINAI REFERENCES

Program Development, Management and Administrative Directions

1950s

Fike N (1957). Social treatment of long-term dependency. *Social Work*, October:51–56.
Goldfarb D, Manko P (1957). Homemaker service in a medical setting. *Children*, 4(6):213–218.
Kozier A (1957). Casework with parents of children born with severe brain defects. *Social Casework*, April.
Siegel D, Knee RI (1959). Unified versus unitized social services in a hospital setting: Issues and implications. *Carnegie Endowment Center Proceedings*. New York:15–29.
Steinberg M, Siegel D (1956). Medical Social Service Necessity or Luxury? *Hospitals*, March 1.
White E (1957). Casework service in a polio respiratory center. *Social Casework*, March.

1960s

Dana B (1965). Health, medical care and social responsibility. *Proceedings 10th Anniversary Symposium: Trends in Practice and Knowledge*. Silver Spring, MD: National Association of Social Workers:57–65.
Gusberg SB, Marinoff S, Hilsen J, Cox L, Young AT, Cameron O (1975). Therapeutic listening: An adolescent guidance program in motivation for contraception. *The Mount Sinai Journal of Medicine*, 42(5):439–444.
Paneth J (1961). Medical social services in the extra-marital pregnancy. *Journal of Jewish Communal Services*, 37(3):270–279.
Rashbaum W, Rehr H, Paneth J, Greenberg, M (1962). Pregnancy in unmarried women, medical and social characteristics. *The Mount Sinai Journal of Medicine*, 30(1):33–45.
Ravich R, Rehr H, Goodrich, C (1969). Ombudsman: a new concept in voluntary hospital services. In WC Richan (Ed.). *Human Services and Social Work Responsibility*. Silver Spring, MD: National Association of Social Workers, Inc.: 311–320.
Ravich R, Rehr H, Goodrich C (1969). Hospital ombudsman smooths flow of services and communication. *Hospitals*, 43:56–61.
Rehr H (1960). Problems for a profession in a strike situation. *Social Work*, 5(2):22–28.
Rehr H, Sauber Mignon (1965). *Hospital Social Services: Analysis of Characteristics and Activities in Servicing the Caseload*. Monograph. New York: The Mount Sinai Hospital, July.
Rehr H, Goodrich C (1969). Problems of innovation in a hospital setting. In WC Richan (Ed.). *Human Services and Social Work Responsibility*. Silver Spring, MD: National Association of Social Workers, 303–309.
Rehr H, Berkman B (1969). Selectivity biases in delivery of hospital social services. *The Social Service Review*, 43(1):35–41.
Rehr H, Berkman B (1967). Aging ward patients and the hospital social service department. *Journal of the American Geriatrics Society*, 15(12):1153–1162.

Rosenfeld E (1968). The therapeutic community-an environment to promote mental health. *Youth Service News, 19*(3):4.

Sauber M, Paneth J (1965). Unwed mothers who keep their children: Research and implications. *Social Work Practice*. New York: Columbia University Press:94–106.

Schonholz D, Gusberg SB, Astrachan JM, Young AT (1969). An adolescent guidance program: Study in education for marital health. *Obstetrics and Gynecology, 34*(4):611–614.

Siegel D (1962). Changing character of the Jewish hospital: Implications for social service administration. *Journal of Jewish Communal Services, 38*(2):282–289.

1970s

Berkman B, Rehr H, Siegel D, Pomrinse D, Paneth J (1971). Utilization of in-patients services by elderly. *Journal of the American Geriatrics Society, 119*(11):933–946.

Berkman B, Rehr H (1973). Early social service casefinding for hospitalized patients: An experiment. *The Social Service Review, 47*(2):256–265.

Berkman B, Rehr H (1973). Social service casefinding in the hospital: Its influence on the utilization of social services. *American Journal of Public Health, 63*(10):857–862.

Berkman B (1978). Mental health and the aging: A review of the literature for clinical social workers. *Clinical Social Work Journal, 6*(3):230–245.

Berkman B (1977). Innovations for delivery of social services in health care. In F Sobey (Ed.). *Changing Roles in Social Work Practice*. Philadelphia, PA: Temple University Press.

Bosch SJ, Merino R, Daniels M, Fischer E, Rosenthal M (1979). A proposed network to improve access to high-quality health care for medicaid-eligible families. *Journal of Community Health, 4*(4):302–311.

Daniels M, Bosch SJ (1978). School health planning: A case for interagency collaboration. *Social Work in Health Care, 3*(4):457–467.

Paneth J (1972). Deflation in an inflationary period: Some current social health need provisions. *American Journal of Public Health, 62*(1):60–63.

Ravich R, Rehr H (1974). Ombudsman program provides feedback. *Hospitals, 48*(18):63–67.

Ravich R (1975). Patient relations. *Hospitals, 49*:(April):3–5.

Rehr H (1972). Mount Sinai's social services in East Harlem now. *Proceedings: A Health Care Plan for East Harlem—Annals of the New York Academy of Sciences, 196*(2):80–81.

Rosenberg G (1977). Cost finding in hospital social work. *Social Work in Health Care, 3*(2):181–186.

Russell TE, Silberman JM (1979). Improving the delivery of specialized foster care services. *Social Casework, 60*(7):402–407.

Siegel D, Rehr H (1971). Evolving social services in psychiatry. *The Mount Sinai Journal of Medicine, 38*(2):185–197.

Wincott E (1976). Comprehensive care: Definitions and a review of selected current delivery models. In *Proceedings Mental Health Services in the Comprehensive Care of the Hemophiliac*, May.

Young AT, Berkman B, Rehr H (1973). Women who seek abortions: A study. *Social Work, 18*(3):60–65.

Young AT, Berkman B, Rehr H (1975). Parental influence on pregnant adolescents. *Social Work, 20*(5):387–391.

1980s

Anvaripour PL, Bernard L, Bronter D, Eden A, Kaplan M, Morris J, Ravich R, Schwartz P (1989). Communicating with hearing impaired patients who utilize the services of a major medical center. *The Journal of the Society of Otorhinolaryngology Head and Neck Surgery*, 7(1):24–26.

Bennett C, Blumenfield S (1989). Enhancing social work practice in health care: a deeper look at behavior in the workplace. *The Clinical Supervisor*, 7(2/3):71–88.

Berkman B, Rehr H, Rosenberg G (1980). A social work department develops and tests a screening mechanism to identify high social risk situations. *Social Work in Health Care*, 5(4):373–385.

Black RB, Weiss JA (1989). Genetic support groups in the development of comprehensive genetic services. *American Journal of Human Genetics*, 45:647–654.

Blumenfield S, Rocklin C (1980). Senior counselor-assistants for a geriatric program in a community hospital. *Social Work in Health Care*, 6(1):89–100.

Blumenfield S, Morris J, Sherman FT (1982). The geriatric team in the acute care hospital: An educational and consultation modality. *Journal of the American Geriatrics Society*, 30(10):660–664.

Blumenfield S (1986). Editorial: Discharge planning: Changes for hospital social work in a new health care climate. *Quality Review Bulletin*, 12(2):51–54.

Blumenfield S, Lowe JI (1987). Data, values and decision-making: A template for analyzing ethical dilemmas in discharge planning. *Health and Social Work*, 12(1):47–56.

Blumenfield S, Rosenberg G (1988). Towards a network of social health services: Redefining discharge planning and expanding the social work domain. *Social Work in Health Care*, 13(4)31–48.

Cantor M, Rehr H, Trotz V (1981). Case management and family involvement. *Mount Sinai Journal of Medicine*, 48(6):566–568.

Clarke S (1983). Hyman J Weiner's use of systems and population approaches. *Social Work in Health Care*, 9(2):5–14.

Clarke S, Neuwirth L, Bernstein R (1986). An expanded social work role in a university hospital-based group practice: Service provider, physician educator and organizational consultant. *Social Work in Health Care*, 11(4):1–18.

Cuzzi L (1985). *Planned Organizational Change in a Department of Social Work*. Dissertation, City University of New York, June.

Daniels M (1980). Social work practice and community health: A planning implementation model. *Social Work in Health Care*, 6(2):39–51.

Dietch HH (1981). Community health ombudsman. In MD Mailick, H Rehr (Eds.). *In the Patient's Interest: Access to Hospital Care*. New York: Prodist:51–66.

Dobrof J (1988). ELAN sets its priorities for the coming year on welfare reform. *Currents of the New York City Chapter of National Association of Social Workers*, November-December:3–4.

Dortz C (1983). Preface. In D Cook, C Fewell, J Riolo (Eds.). *Social Work Treatment of Alcohol Problems*. Piscataway, NJ: Rutgers Center Alcohol Studies: IX–XI.

Fischel-Wolovick L, Cotter C, Masser I, Kelman-Bravo E, Jaffe RS, Rosenberg G, Wittenberg B (1988). Alternative work scheduling for professional social workers. *Administration in Social Work*, 12(4):93–102.

Genkins M (1985). Strategic planning for social work marketing. *Administration in Social Work*, 9(1):35–46.

Genkins M (1986). *Marketing Theory: Applicability to Social Work Service in Health Care Delivery.* Dissertation, City University of New York.

Gordon N (1982). *Organizational Change in a Medical Setting: A Field Work Curriculum for Direct Practice Students.* Dissertation, City University of New York.

Gruber T (1980). The Pre-admission Screening Process. In DR Heacock (Ed.). *A Psychodynamic Approach to Adolescent Psychiatry: The Mount Sinai Experience.* New York: Marcel Dekker, Inc.:15–23.

Haber-Scharf M (1985). Costing social work services in a hospital setting. *Social Work in Health Care,*11(1):113–129.

Jacobs P, Lurie A, Cuzzi L (1980). Coordination of services to methadone mothers and their addicted newborns. *Health and Social Work,* 8(4):290–298.

Krell GI, Rosenberg G (1983). Predicting patterns of social work staffing in hospital settings. *Social Work in Health Care,* 9(2):61–79.

Levy LP (1982). The integration of the foster grandparent program with an acute care psychiatric service. *Social Work in Health Care,* 8(1):27–35.

Lewis M (1988). Caregiving: An emerging health issue. Monograph. *America Meets Australia: Alzheimer's Disease—Researching the Questions.* South Melbourne, Australia.

Lipsky H, Sherman F (1984). Case study K—the geriatric evaluation and treatment service. In SJ Brody, NA Persily (Eds.). *Hospital and the Aged.* Rockville, MD: Aspen Systems Corp:219–225.

Lurie A, Rosenberg G (Eds.). (1984). *Social Work Administration in Health Care.* New York: Haworth Press.

Mailick M, Rehr H (Eds.). (1981). *In the Patient's Interest: Access to Hospital Care.* New York: Prodist.

Mailick MD (1981). The current climate. In MD Mailick, H Rehr (Eds.). *In the Patient's Interest: Access to Hospital Care.* New York: Prodist:17–30.

Mailick MD (1981). Models of patient representative programs. In MD Mailick, H Rehr (Eds.). *In the Patient's Interest: Access to Hospital Care.* New York: Prodist: 85–111.

Mailick MD (1981). Professionals view patient representatives. In MD Mailick, H Rehr (Eds.). *In the Patient's Interest: Access to Hospital Care.* New York: Prodist: 112–129.

Mailick MD (1982). Patient representative programs: A social work perspective. *Social Work in Health Care,* 7(4):39–51.

Mailick MD (1983). The ombudsman in health care institutions in the United States. In G Caiden (Ed.). *International Handbook of the Ombudsman: Evaluation and Present Function.* Westport, CT: Greenwood Press:121–128.

Mailick MD (1984). Steps to professionalization: patient representatives. *Journal of Allied Health,* November:263–270.

Mailick MD, Jordan P (1989). A multi-model approach to collaborative practice. In K Davidson, S Clarke (Eds.). *Social Work in Health Care.* New York: Haworth Press:295–307.

McKinney E, Young AT (1985). Changing patient populations: Considerations for service delivery. *Health and Social Work,* 10(4):292–299.

Miller RS, Rehr H (Eds.) (1983). *Social Work Issues in Health Care.* Englewood Cliffs, NJ: Prentice-Hall, Inc.

Morrison B, Rehr H, Rosenberg G, Davis S (1982). Consumer opinion surveys: A hospital quality assurance measurement. *Quality Review Bulletin,* 8(2):19–24.

Pianko L, Sherman F, Rehr H, Sacks H (1981). Acceptance of pneumococcal vaccination by the community residing elderly. *The Geronotologist, 21*:240–241.

Ravich R (1981). The society of patient representatives. In MD Mailick, H Rehr (Eds.). *In the Patient's Interest: Access to Hospital Care.* New York: Prodist:130–145.

Ravich R, Weissman GK (1981). Revised discharge form improves continuity of care. *The Hospital Medical Staff, 10*(2):12–19.

Ravich R (1986). Patient advocacy. In J Marks (Ed.). *Advocacy in Health Care.* Clifton, NJ: Humana Press:51–60.

Rehr H, Elster S (Eds.) (1981). Geriatrics and gerontology: A multi-disciplinary approach to medical and social problems. *Mount Sinai Journal of Medicine, 48*(6): 478,575–577.

Rehr H (1981). Access to services: A complex dimension. In MD Mailick, H Rehr (Eds.). *In the Patient's Interest: Access to Hospital Care.* New York: Prodist: 1–10.

Rehr H, Ravich R (1981). An ombudsman in the hospital: The patient representative. In MD Mailick, H Rehr (Eds.). *In the Patient's Interest: Access to Hospital Care.* New York: Prodist:68–84.

Rehr H, Mailick M (Eds.) (1981). Dilemmas, conclusions and recommendations. In *The Patient's Interest: Access to Hospital Care.* New York: Prodist:146–171.

Rehr H (1981). The patient representative: A facilitator of services in the general hospital. *Information and Referral: Journal of the Alliance of Information and Referral Systems, 3*(1):1–19.

Rehr H (1983). More issues for the eighties. In RS Miller, H Rehr (Eds.). *Social Work Issues in Health Care.* Englewood Cliffs, NJ: Prentice-Hall:252–277.

Rehr H (1984). Health care and social work services: Present and future concerns and directions. *Social Work in Health Care, 10*(1):71–83.

Rehr H (1986). Social work in health care for the eighties. In B Berkman (Ed.). *Social Work in Health Care Lectures*, MGH Institute of Health Professions. Boston, MA: MGH.

Rehr H (Ed.) (1986). *Access to Social-health Care: Who Shall Decide What?* Lexington, MA: Ginn Press.

Rehr H, Rosenberg G (1986). Access to social health care: Implication for social work. In H Rehr (Ed.) *Access to Social-health Care: Who Shall Decide What?* Lexington, MA:Ginn Press:77–96.

Rosenberg G (1980). Concepts in the financial management of hospital social work departments. *Social Work in Health Care, 5*(3)287–297. Also in A Lurie, G Rosenberg (Eds.). *Social Work Administration in Health Care.* New York: Haworth Press:131–141.

Rosenberg G, Weissman A (1981). Marketing social services in health care facilities. *Health and Social Work, 6*(3):13–20. Also in A Lurie, G Rosenberg (Eds.), *Social Work Administration in Health Care.* New York: Haworth Press:259–270.

Rosenberg G, Rehr H (Eds.) (1983). *Advancing Social Work Practice in the Health Care Field: Emerging Issues and New Perspectives.* New York: Haworth Press.

Rosenberg G (1984). The author responds—to Patricia Volland. In A Lurie, G Rosenberg (Eds.). *Social Work Administration in Health Care.* New York: Haworth Press:146–147.

Rosenberg G, Speedling E, Rehr H, Morrison B (1985). Some effects of a hospital employee strike on patient satisfaction. *The Mount Sinai Journal of Medicine, 52*(4):259–264.

Rosenberg G (1986). Social work in the future: Predictions and strategies. *Current Issues in Health Care for Professional Leaders: Problems and Potentials and Changes in Health Care: A Challenge to the Profession.* Monograph. New York: Columbia University School of Social Work:May 20:35–46.

Rosenberg G, Clarke S (Eds.) (1987). *Social Workers in Health Care Management: The Move to Leadership.* New York: Haworth Press.

Rosenberg G, Clarke S (1987). The study: Purpose and method. In G Rosenberg, S Clarke (Eds.). *Social Workers in Health Care Management: The Move to Leadership.* New York: Haworth Press:1–4.

Rosenberg G, Clarke (1987). The social worker as manager in health care settings: An experiential view. In G Rosenberg, S Clarke (Eds.). *Social Workers in Health Care Management: The Move to Leadership.* New York: Haworth Press:71–84.

Rosenberg G, Clarke S (1987). Findings and implications. In G Rosenberg, S Clarke (Eds.). *Social Workers in Health Care Management: The Move to Leadership.* New York: Haworth Press:143–159.

Rosenberg G, Dana B (1989). Social implications of health care in contemporary perspectives: Essays in honor of Helen Rehr. *Mount Sinai Journal of Medicine, 56*(6):427–428.

Rosengarten L (1986). Creating a health-promoting group for elderly couples on a home health care program. *Social Work in Health Care, 11*(4):83–92.

Rosengarten L (1989). Case management: A definition in historical perspective. *Issues in Service Coordination for the Elderly with Developmental Disabilities (Unit 5, Module 5, Aging and Developmental Disabilities: A Training Inservice Package),* 8–21.

Speedling E, Morrison B, Rehr H, Rosenberg G (1983). Patient satisfaction: Closing the gap between provider and consumer. *Quality Review Bulletin, 9*(8):224–228.

Speedling E, Rosenberg G (1986). Patient well-being: A responsibility for hospital managers. *Health Care Management Review, 11*(3):9–19.

Speedling E, McDermott M, Eichhorn S, Rosenberg G (1987). Hospital employee-patient relations: A program for enhancing patient well-being. *Hospital and Health Services Administration,* February:71–82.

Walther V (1983). Commentary on John Wax's clinical contributions to administration practice. In G Rosenberg, H Rehr (Eds.). *Advancing Social Work Practice in the Health Care Field.* New York: Haworth Press:142–145. Also in *Social Work in Health Care, 8*(3).

Walther V (1986). Changes in health care today: A challenge to the maternal and child health services social workers. In *Changes in Health Care Today: A Challenge to the Profession.* Monograph. New York: Columbia University School of Social Work:79–84.

Weissman A (1986). Linkage in Direct Practice. *Encyclopedia of Social Work,* 8th Edition. Silver Spring, MD: National Association of Social Workers, Inc.:47–50.

Weissman A (1989). A social worker comments: Quality referrals. *Social Work in Health Care, 13*(1):51–56.

1990s

Belville R, Indyk D, Shapiro V, *et al.* (1991). The community as a strategic site for refining high perinatal risk assessments and interventions. *Social Work in Health Care, 16*(1):5–19.

Bernstein SR (1991). Contracted Services: Issues for the Non-profit Agency Manager. *Sector Quality, 22*(4):429–443.

Bernstein SR (1991). *Managing Contracted Services in the Non-profit Agency: Administrative Ethical and Political Issues.* Philadelphia, PA: Temple University Press.

Black RB, Weiss JA (1990). Genetic support groups and social workers as partners. *Health and Social Work, 15*(2):91–99.

Black RB (1991). Social work practice with children and adolescents with chronic illness and disabilities. In S Bardfield, RG Black (Eds.). *Social Work Practice With Maternal and Child Health: Populations at Risk, A Casebook.* New York: Columbia University School of Social Work:165–173.

Davidson KW, Clarke S (Eds.) (1990). *Social Work in Health Care: A Handbook for Practice* (Two Volumes). New York: Haworth Press.

Dobrof J, Umpierre M, Rocha L, Silverton M (1990). Group work in a primary care medical setting. *Health and Social Work, 15*(1):32–37.

Eichhorn S, Speedling E, Rosenberg G (1991). Changing the way we work. *The Health Care Forum Journal, 34*(2):45–48.

Mailick MD (1991). Editorial: Recruitment and retention of MSW graduates. *Social Work in Health Care, 16*(2):1–4.

Mason J, Preisinger J, Sperling R, Walther V, Berrier, J, Evans V (1991). Incorporating HIV education and counseling into routine prenatal care. *AIDS Education and Prevention, 3*(2):118–123.

Rehr H (1990). Discharge planning: An ongoing function of quality care. *Quality Review Bulletin, 12*:(February):47–50.

Rehr H (1991). Integrating practice and research. In C Irizarry, C James (Eds.). *Achieving Excellence in Health Social Work.* Adelaide, Australia: Flinders Press:54–84.

Rehr H (1991). High social-risk screening. In C Irizarry, C James (Eds.). *Achieving Excellence in Health Social Work.* Adelaide, Australia: Flinders Press:97–126.

Rehr H (1991). The state of affairs in health social work. In C Irizarry, C James (Eds.). *Achieving Excellence in Health Social Work.* Adelaide, Australia: Flinders Press:9–25.

Rehr H, Rosenberg G (Eds.) (1991). *The Changing Context of Social-health Care: Its Implications for Providers and Consumers.* New York: Haworth Press.

Rosengarten L, Rosengarten F (1990). Aspects of cooperative home care for the elderly in Bologna, Italy. *Pride Institute Journal of Long-term Home Health Care, 9*:32–37.

Schwartz P, Blumenfield S, Simon EP (1990). The interim homecare program: An innovative discharge planning alternative. *Health and Social Work, 15*(2):152–160.

Simon EP (1990). The therapeutic companion program. *Archives of the Foundation of Thanatology, 16*(2).

Simon EP (1991). Interim home care meet both patients and hospital needs. *Picker/Commonwealth Report, 1*:(Spring):7–8.

Stein E, Wade K, Smith D (1991). Clinical support groups that work. *Journal of the Association of Nurses in AIDs Care (Janac), 2*(2):29–36.

Young AT (1991). Social work practice with adolescent health and teenage pregnancy. In S Bardfield, B Black (Eds.). *Social Work Practice with Maternal and Child Health: Populations at Risk, A Casebook.* New York: Columbia University School of Social Work:17–25.

5

Professional Accountability and Quality Improvement Through Practice-Based Studies

Helen Rehr, Nancy Showers, Alma Young, and Susan Blumenfield

"To be professional is to be accountable, to be answerable to someone or to some group, to possess full and complete information upon which to make decisions, decisions that are judgments relating to a program, a population, a group, or a patient and his family. In professional terms accountability is the capacity and capability to assume responsibility for those acts and behaviors undertaken to achieve identified [sic] objectives. A key characteristic of a profession is that it, through its members, sets standards for its members' practice. Another is that it, again through its members, monitors professional services, correcting where necessary and, in general, advancing the quality of all" (Rehr, 1979; p. 150).

Accountability is professional only when professionals are involved in making it so. Although supported by the institution or agency, social workers are individually accountable. Each seeks to provide quality service and to improve client services on an ongoing basis. A self-directed worker is one who assumes professional accountability as he looks to quality assurance measures in continually assessing services and improving the quality of care. Quality is a multidimensional term that encompasses many factors, such as appropriate decision making, effectiveness, access, environmental safety, continuity of care, and qualitative interactions between client and clinician (O'Leary, 1991; p. 72). Professionals must be accountable for their performance and programs across these dimensions. "The final payoff is outcomes" (O'Leary, p. 74).

Measures of performance relate to the individual's condition, provider performance and interventions, and a "sound infrastructure of care" (O'Leary, 1995) as well as to individual attitudes and beliefs. The objective of evaluation is to measure practice, performance, and outcomes and determine if changes in performance and standards of care are necessary. Quality assurance (QA) addresses the quality of programs and their capacity to meet the rules, regulations, and expectations of accrediting bodies.

BACKGROUND

Florence Nightingale first introduced the concept of quality assessment in the 1860s. Flexner (1925) reviewed medical care in the United States and first reported on its deficiencies in 1910. Both of their efforts precipitated major changes in medical and nursing education, and in their practice. In 1912, (DHEW, 1977) Codman attempted to assess the end result of hospital care, asking what medicine does and what are the outcomes of its practice. His review of surgical outcomes in hospitals led to the Hospital Standardization Program of the American College of Surgeons in 1918, which was precursor to accreditation standards, patient care evaluation, and outcomes measurement concepts. In 1951, the American College of Surgeons joined with other major medical professions and associations to form the Joint Commission on the Accreditation of Hospitals (since 1986, the Joint Commission on the Accreditation of Health Organizations). JCAHO became the nation's voluntary accrediting body, developing standards and surveying and accrediting hospitals and other health care institutions based on those standards.

Patient care evaluation in medical institutions had a slow start. By and large, activities were lodged in internal medical peer review committees that set their own guidelines and judged practice, protecting the institution and the professions from outside review. In 1965, the enactment of Titles 18 and 19 of the Social Security Act mandated what previously had been a voluntary process of quality and professional review. By 1972, PL 92-603 established professional review organizations and crystallized requirements for evaluation of the quality of medical care. Soon quality assurance requirements for medical care became central to the agenda of every federal, state, and national regulatory agency, including JCAHO.

In the 1970s little was known about the extent of health services available and who received them. Internally derived data were not shared among institutions, let alone used to enhance regional services. What little was known was believed to be an institution's or department's private preserve. Federal demand for utilization review and public accountability changed that belief, and many felt their autonomy threatened. Like other health care professionals, many social workers viewed the requirement for professional accountability as a political attack on their services, while others sought the greater professional status they believed it would help them achieve.

CONTINUOUS QUALITY IMPROVEMENT

By the 1990s, the JCAHO's evaluation requirements had evolved to focus on a new process—that of continuous quality improvement (CQI). CQI calls for a system of continuous self-examination of institutional and provider practice in defined areas, such as the performance of the individual as a self-directed practitioner, and the collective action of the team unit or system. CQI is an expectation held by consumers, providers, institutions, payers, and regulators, and those in the community-at-large.

The CQI process focuses on improving outcomes for patients and populations while incorporating patients' views of those outcomes. CQI is a collaborative process that engages doctors and other health care professionals and that seeks to improve professional performance and systems of care without being punitive. For social work in health care, CQI is one means to further integrate medical and nonmedical services. Medical services and other social-health services have been translated into indicators that cover accessibility, availability, comprehensiveness, coordination of care, the utilization of personnel, safety, and patient and provider attitudes toward care. Individual adherence to standards of practice is explored as well as the extent of patient education. Other outcome measures address consumer and provider satisfaction with services. The quality of provider commitment to care, change, and continuing education also are measured.

The benefits of this continuous and collaborative process should provide patients and their families with more comprehensive care, physicians and other health care professionals with more informed data regarding their patients, and the institution with improved utilization of services. Integration of these systems can improve access to services and their coordination. Improvement in efficiency should lead to cost-effectiveness.

CONTINUOUS QUALITY IMPROVEMENT
IN SOCIAL WORK SERVICES

For social work, effective CQI leads to clinical planning and improvement, providing opportunities to review who is being served, what services they are getting, and whether the best clinical care possible is being given. Although CQI studies address groups of patients, they are seen through individual study. Thus programs can be assessed for their benefits, and assessment can serve as a key to patient individualization. This approach has allowed social workers to standardize guidelines for high social-risk screening and introduce early casefinding methods.

Is casework effective? Some in social work suggest it is not possible to answer the question (Briar 1980). Others (Doherty & Streeter, 1993; Thomlinson, 1984) have demonstrated that clients cite beneficial results. Health settings not only are systems for care delivery but also serve as "a living laboratory for research" (Berkman, 1975). Both scientific and applied studies occur in most medical institutions on an ongoing basis. Social workers are exposed to and involved in "ongoing research of the medical and psychiatric departments, hospital administration, the regulatory agencies, and their own social work departments" (Berkman & Weissman, 1983; p. 221). They are expected to evaluate the services they deliver.

COMPLEXITIES OF EVALUATION

Evaluation of care is complex. It is difficult to know the direct relationship of the problem to process and to outcome. No unilinear theory or relationship supports such a paradigm. Nor does any service outcome evolve from the total autonomy of a clinician. Clients can present simple or complex problems that might be perceived differently by different providers. Client interventions can be as diverse as those based on extant theoretical formulations or on the art of practice. Outcome, which is difficult to measure, might be intertwined with many intervening variables that make it difficult to establish a cause-intervention effect. Outcome reviews of social work services by researchers have not always supported positive results. The findings of Fischer (1978) and Wood (1978) on effectiveness might well reflect the concern with major social ills, such as delinquency or poverty. As social workers examined issues related to social-environmental ailments, they tended to overlook the benefits of applied studies. Lawlor and Raube (1995) note, ". . . there is growing acknowledgment that the frontier problems of health service delivery involve considerable social service and public health content, where the conditioning of human behavior is more important than medical technique and where the critical venue of care is in community settings, not in hospitals" (p. 400). Social workers need "to realize that the etiology of social ailments is lodged in a complex mosaic [which requires] a multidisciplinary approach to goal formulation and treatment direction, an approach to which social work can contribute" (*Research on Social Work Practice*, 1992) to broad societal policy deliberations.

TYPES OF STUDIES

Social work services are not based on an exact science. No set rules exist for a given performance related to specific problems. Practice is prescribed by expectations in the clinical process addressing entry and assessment skills, diagnosis, contracting with clients, interventive and collaborative skills, and ultimately outcomes (Rosenberg, 1983). These are eclectic and very much lodged in Schon's (1983) reflection-in-action. Practice studies are essential professional accountability measures aimed at informing practice and improving performance and program. Studies can be descriptive, process-oriented, related to satisfaction with care by clients and providers, and/or they can review the effectiveness of achieving client and program goals. Social workers in health care settings have drawn on all of these study methods to review and assure the quality of care (Berkman & Weissman, 1983).

EPIDEMIOLOGICAL METHODS

Epidemiological methods have served social workers as they review population groups and their needs. Mega-analysis has become an important research tool in which to review multiple comparable studies to understand population groups. Benchmarking has permitted social work administrators to compare their department's performance with that of comparable departments and institutions. Such administrative studies validate social work services within the institution, demonstrate their effectiveness, facilitate management and improvement, and increase visibility to hospital administration, the board, health care providers, regulatory agencies, and even the community.

THE RELEVANT LITERATURE

The field of social work had anticipated the involvement of and impact on its own profession of quality assurance requirements and had begun, without mandate, to evolve toward its own assessment of practice and performance. In the more than 30 years since it first identified the need to study the quality of patient care and services, the department of social work services has kept pace with changes in requirements for QA activities, as a leader in its own profession and within the institution. By 1972, the department was participating in independent studies, having recognized the need to review service utilization patterns and patient needs, beginning with its experience during the poliomyelitis epidemic of the 1950s and early 1960s.

OBJECTIVES FOR STUDY

Creation of an academic division of social work brought a formal commitment to engage in collaborative research with other health care professionals. The research section of the division, supported by the department of social work services, whose practices and programs were the source of those studies, set objectives to:

- undertake applied social work research relevant to and functional for the development and the enhancement of social work services; and
- enhance the delivery of social and health service by affecting the social and psychological milieu of the setting and of its providers.

From the mid-1950s on, a climate was set for study. As social workers reviewed their practice, they attempted to assess structure, process, and outcomes through small applied studies. They sought to advance knowledge and effective skills derived from the study programs and performance, and from review and feedback to themselves as practitioners. Feedback demonstrated that studies were relevant to practice, based on the questions such studies evoked, and critical for the quality and enhancement of practice.

PRACTICE-BASED STUDIES

Social work staff used practice-based studies as the primary means of evaluation. They ventured across a wide field from early audits, standard setting, and achievements—guaranteeing access, program, and performance assessments, and cost-effective care delivery in terms of outcomes and consumer and provider satisfaction with care. Their early studies were referred to as "one-page research" in which the practicing social worker identified a single question with a few variables based on her observations. Using these variables, social workers examined patient-family cases for answers. When a question crossed a number of workers' paths or when the issues were greater than a single question, study findings were looped back to practitioners to improve their practice and to recommend change in structure and/or program where indicated.

Research ideas were and are generated from discussions by social work practitioners of what they do, with whom and how, and what happens.

Group discussions facilitate quality improvement in either program or performance, the essence of professional accountability. The one-page approach helps demystify research and assist workers to ask key questions, such as "what do I want to know?" Group discussion, sometimes with technical research assistance, helps the social worker translate the question into doable segments. The methodology involves building blocks of small-scale studies that might lead to broader-based research.

THE RELEVANT LITERATURE

SOCIAL AND PHYSICAL FUNCTIONING

In the 1950s and early 1960s the medical and social services that might affect the social and physical functioning rehabilitation of severe polio victims were reviewed. These studies resulted in enhanced programs that took comprehensive care into the homes of the polio patients and provided support to patients' families.

ACCESS TO SERVICES

In the same time period social workers and obstetricians sought ways to curb repeat pregnancies in unwed teenagers. Studies asked, who were these pregnant girls? What was their use of medical and social services? and Who kept their babies? The findings uncovered wide cultural diversity and disparity of available resources related to that diversity, which led to changes in social-health care delivery to teenage pregnant girls and enhanced networking with community facilities. A program of adolescent guidance with health education was introduced and monitored. Collaboration and team services are widely evidenced in these programs.

THE ELDERLY'S UTILIZATION OF SERVICES

Social work, with hospital administration, examined the elderly's utilization of institutional services, learning that indigent patients served in the old wards and those served in semiprivate and private rooms posed similar problems. Irrespective of social class, elderly patients required similar resources during their posthospital care. The resources were differentiated only by people's ability to pay for what was available. When the Medicare and Medicaid legislation was introduced, social work was serving all of the sick elderly referred for service. But studies of the timeliness of social service entry as a result of referrals showed that those with serious needs reached social work services too late (if at all) in the hospital stay to ensure adequate discharge planning. These studies of the casefinding system of referrals were advanced into the 1970s and led to standards for guaranteeing access to care (Vourlekis, 1990).

PATIENT REPRESENTATIVE AND SOCIAL-HEALTH ADVOCACY

Obstacles included not only lack of needed services but also fragmented services, barriers, or closed doors. As a result of study, the department pioneered an ombudsman program, in which patient representatives could advocate for patients; and a social-health advocate program that assisted local, low-income patients to secure entitlements. Both programs continue to this day. Patient representative programs have become institutionalized and recognized by the American Hospital Association.

The patient representative program has continued to study problems, and as problems are identified it reports them to appropriate department chiefs. Changes are made to accommodate people more efficiently. A number of patient-oriented instruments were tested during the 1980s. An information pamphlet on discharge is now offered to patients to help initiate the social worker-patient relationship in ambulatory care. An immediately available simple discharge form overcomes the common obstacle of medical chart availability in the clinic, and safeguards continuity of care. As greater coordination of care is introduced, fragmentation has been reduced. The patient representative program serves all those who encounter obstacles to or have complaints about care in the hospital. The social-health advocacy program helps hospitalized patients who require referral services.

In the late 1980s, REAP (resource, entitlement, advocacy program), a social work service program established by the institution, was stationed as a storefront satellite across from the hospital and is open to anyone who needs help with their entitlements or with referral to services.

A SOCIAL-HEALTH MODEL

The work of the 1960s produced a social-health model of services, because studies reflected the need to integrate principles of individualization and social-health care into the existing biomedical model. Federal QA legislation challenged the department to become accountable in a formal sense. Early studies concentrated on who was served, where, and for what. As social workers interpreted findings, impediments to good, socially oriented care were uncovered and patient-family social-health needs were defined.

CASEFINDING SYSTEM PIONEERED

In the 1970s, social workers furthered the autonomy of social work services. By demonstrating the extent of social need through clinical indicators of high social and medical risk and uncovering problematic compliance with recommendations, social work pioneered its own casefinding system. The system of high social-risk screening could be introduced at preadmission or soon after admission when patient/family risk for return to home could be identified, and predictions made for support and assistance and the need for early intervention. Using epidemiological methods, social workers introduced studies of those at-risk for social problems. Early casefinding of high social-risk elderly led to reductions in length-of-stay, cost-containment, and quality aftercare planning. As studies uncovered the most vulnerable patients and family members, it became clear that dependence on other health professionals for referral resulted in inappropriate utilization of social services.

HIGH SOCIAL-RISK SCREENING, CASEFINDING, AND SATISFACTION STUDIES

During the 1980s, studies refined high social-risk screening and casefinding methods. These studies were epidemiologically based with a view toward analyzing the needs of selected population groups. As workers learned what works and what does not, they advanced social-risk screening into new arenas, such as the preadmission screening of elderly patients awaiting elective surgery. Although the particular study gleaned positive patient response about their posthospital arrangements, it was less cost-effective than at-admission screening. Even though preadmission screening seemed more costly, the findings helped social workers and administrators learn that early quality approaches to patients were meaningful. Studies prompted application of early high social-risk screening as a standard measure for professional accountability by social work departments across the country.

Patient satisfaction studies have been constantly refined to become routine quality improvement instruments, and their findings are used to improve services. Satisfaction studies focused on the consumer and the range of services received. Clinical indicators are a standard in continuous quality improvement. As quarterly surveys are reviewed, findings are shared with hospital middle managers and members of the board of trustees to keep them informed about the quality of care. Satisfaction studies substantiated a high positive correlation between client and worker perceptions of services. Professional accountability was demonstrated as study findings led to enhanced access to services, evaluation and refinement of services and programs, and introduction of new standards to ensure the relevance, efficiency, and effectiveness of social services.

SOCIAL-HEALTH PROBLEM CLASSIFICATION

To study the effectiveness of social services, a social-health problem classification was developed and validated. Problem classification enabled social workers to undertake the resolution of problem-related services, and a telephone follow-up system helped social workers learn whether clients were satisfied with the outcomes of care.

COLLABORATIVE EFFORTS

In the 1980s, joint efforts by physicians and social workers addressed patient response to the introduction of selected drugs in a range of inpatients suffering from different mental illnesses; these efforts proved beneficial to both professions in serving these patients. Psychoeducational models of care also were analyzed. Another study demonstrated a relationship between psychopathology and menstruation. If those symptoms were to be described today they might be evaluated in a biological context rather than in the psychopathologic context prevalent in the early 1980s.

Women who evidenced sterilization regrets were studied, and a counseling program was developed for those seeking sterilization. The introduction of genetics counseling for selected patients was undertaken, and its outcomes reviewed. Concurrently, the genetics specialists studied physicians' knowledge of Tay Sachs, a somewhat rare disease, and introduced content into continuing medical education programs.

Education for health care professionals at the student and practitioner levels became a critical factor in advancing quality performance. Social work reviewed student knowledge and skills to determine learning needs and offer guidelines. An instrument to assess social work education in the medical setting was developed. Students' satisfaction with the educational experience was reviewed. They gave high marks to the field experience and hands-on learning under the supervision of skilled practitioners.

At the end of the 1970s, a comparative analysis among affiliated institutions of their patterns of medical and social components in patient care was completed. Their implications were projected for the education of all health care professionals with particular emphasis on the value of multi-professional collaboration.

AREAS FOR CONTINUED STUDY

The cost-effectiveness of social services has been correlated with efficient and available delivery of care. In an early approach to setting standards for coverage, the social work field in health care attempted to examine staffing needs for hospitals with different bed capacities. Now because such vast new technology has been introduced, hospitalization has become more selective, and ambulatory care more evident forcing a reassessment of staffing patterns. Understanding who are at high social risk will continue to be studied as it relates to staffing patterns. The basis for staffing patterns will be severity of illness, chronic disability and the degree of physical and social functioning limitations, a patient's motivation for self-care, and individual and family ability to support their needs as well as availability of more formal networks in the community. The loci of social services will expand to include arenas beyond the institutional walls in which the vulnerable receive care.

As social workers studied their cases, they found that family members need to be more directly involved in patient care and more involved with the patients' doctors. Contracting with patients and family members has been given primary attention as workers examine the outcome of services.

SUBSTANCE ABUSE

Social workers demonstrated their roles in a range of studies addressing adolescents and children involved in substance abuse. They developed instruments to study behavior and its predictability. Techniques of meta-analysis were used to review multiple published studies for intrinsic findings. Studies were undertaken in a wide range of client populations.

CONCLUSION

Is social work improving the social-health status of its clients and potential clients? Is social work systematically improving the delivery of care and advancing toward the best care possible? Is it offering the most cost-effective programs? These questions hinge on answers gained through systematic approaches to CQI through applied studies that draw on a framework of clinical indicators of service (Vourlekis, 1990s), more formal evaluations of care, and biomedically and sociologically based scientific studies that test hypotheses.

As they study their performance and programs, either social work-specific or shared with other health care professionals, the focus of health care social work practitioners is on how their performance and programs will affect clients. Their responsiveness to study derives from observation and from doing. Theirs is an inductive process based on knowledge, experience, and intuition which lead to reflection and to action (Schon, 1983).

As social workers reflect on their individual cases, they seek to understand what they observed in the client's situation and what they contributed to the institution that led to change. As they reflect on their cases in the collective, they must recognize the implications of their interventions and those of other providers for program enhancement. Their interests have led to studies that examine social work practice and its effectiveness, the social-environmental connection to medical care and health maintenance, and the service and program impediments that fragment and limit patient care. Studies about client satisfaction with care in general and with social work services in particular have led to important changes in practice and programs.

In developing a framework for quality assessment, social workers formulated the department's objectives clearly. As new programs were piloted, the basic underlying premise called for professional accountability which workers translated to mean in-house studies of performance and programs. Such studies were essential to improving and supporting quality service. The key focus of social work study has been on patients' and families' social and health risk in the hospital, at home, in their community environment, and in their interrelationships with those who affect their health status. Social workers have viewed the at-risk concept in the context of individuals' social functioning within their physical status in their own environment. This concept has affected multidisciplinary practice and its study as psychosocial-environmental factors have been introduced into diagnosis and treatment and the study of disease and disability. In the institution, patterns of patient utilization and satisfaction with services have uncovered deterrents to comprehensive and coordinated services, which have led the administration to change staff routines and programs, thus serving as clinical indicators in reviewing quality care in social work accountability.

Although neither practitioners nor researchers can offer a uniform approach to the extant psychotherapies or psychosocial treatment and their merit, for those who provide such services to clientele, observations and experiences lead to specifics for inquiry governing these questions. One of the clinical values of study is to offer the practitioner the opportunity to understand better, have information for assessment and treatment, and learn the outcome of service. For information to be beneficial, it needs to support monitoring and ultimately improve care. "From the public's point of view, there are two major conceptual areas of interest, health care in general and perceived personal health status. In health care the object of measurement is the system, its structure, and its processes. Under health status, it is the public's perception of personal health outcomes (e.g., functioning, well-being)" (Ware, 1995; p. 25).

Individual clinicians have always been involved in a process of gathering and analyzing data which determines the interventions and course of psychosocial treatment. By extending the exercise to wider phenomena (i.e., to groups of patients or clusters of problems or interventions), the clinician becomes a researcher (Blumenfield, 1993; p. 1). In addition, a host of reasons exist to invest in professional review of services: assessment of the clinical performance of individual practitioners to contribute to the development of practice knowledge and ongoing skills; assessment of the quality of clinical programs and their need for improvement; knowledge of client satisfaction with services received and provider satisfaction with services delivered; determination of the need for continuing education; determination of problems in access to care; identification of internal expertise for consultation purposes. These reasons lead to projections for basic social work education.

The pursuit of professional accountability called for a partnership between practitioners and administration. Such a partnership supports the belief that performance and program need to be reviewed periodically and that opportunities for open discussion and for sharing frustrations, questions, and ideas need to be available. Shared power and decision making are the tools for examination and change. Practitioners can make significant contributions and have done so. They know their practice settings and how to negotiate them. They transpose findings readily into practice and program.

The approach that served the department and worked well in study and application was to:

- diagnose the problem together through open communication;
- set objectives mutually;
- use a participatory approach involving open interventions and reaching group consensus;
- disseminate the maximum information available (not the least);
- invest all participants in the process;

- discuss findings for implications;
- discuss findings for recommendations, implementation of change, and role assignments;
- disseminate change recommendations and implement the training required; and
- invest in a periodic review of changes and continued open discussion (Rehr, 1992; p. 253).

The practitioner and the researcher have similar responsibilities: each is expected to give a logical account of what she has done. Both must document their successes and failures. To this end, social work must integrate research into practice, and researchers must relate to the art of practice. It is critical to study outcomes in the social-health status of individuals and groups. If one considers that the critical outcomes of health care are in an individual's behavior and social and physical functioning, then outcomes research allows practitioners and researchers to find common ground.

Outcomes research or "medical effectiveness research" appears to reflect that many health care problems are primarily social, not medical, in nature (Lawlor & Raube, 1995; p. 383). This means of study has "developed specific packages of outcomes that are appropriate for given diagnostic or problem identification" (p. 398). A set of indicators can range over a number of outcomes, such as "changes in functional status [activities of daily living and instrumental activities of daily living]; health status signs and symptoms; knowledge, demonstrated skill, and compliance; family/caregiver stress; unmet needs; satisfaction; and use of services" (p. 398). Outcome measures can serve as the expectation of specific provider assignment. By setting guidelines for social-health care interventions against given problems, one can ask "what works effectively?" The standards and guidelines require the expertise of many disciplines—the integration of "social science, public health and medicine" (p. 401)—so as to test "the effectiveness of health services that involve medical and nonmedical interventions and outcomes" (p. 401).

Outcomes research is thus a quality measure reflecting on the integration of theory and experience. The social costs of health policies and programs, particularly how they affect the sick in the hospital environment and the well-being of those in the community, are also essential areas of study in the context of cost-effectiveness or outcomes of given programs, as well as the lack of service. Thus social workers must not only conduct applied studies of their own services but also participate in collaborative studies with other health care professionals and consumer groups.

The professions must commit themselves again to the public good. Continuous quality improvement is, in our opinion, synonymous with professional accountability; which is a fundamental issue in public policy, and valued as a social contract between the public and the health care professional. Quality improvement goes beyond standard setting to evaluating performance and program, learning the who and what of populations being served and to be served. It provides information for coordinating care, conducting population at-risk studies, making clinical decisions, and relating to the financial elements of service and planning. As social workers reflect on their practice, they are "researchers" of practice. They study *in* rather than *on* practice.

Small-scale studies inform and help to underpin clinical know-how, as they empower the social worker. They help every health care professional commit to a lifetime of building professional knowledge and delivering the best services available. By reviewing the publications of practice per se, researchers may find clinically relevant findings that are visibly meaningful to those delivery services. Social work practice and academia will need practice-research consortia, a federation of agreeing parties in given regions that sets an organizational climate for study. It is more than consultation; rather it is a partnership wherein practice sets the agenda in which relevant study serves the public good (Epstein, 1995). In addition, as participants with other health care professionals in outcome and/or effectiveness research and in deliberating social-health policy, social workers will contribute to positive outcomes of social-health services to individuals and groups.

MOUNT SINAI REFERENCES

PROFESSIONAL ACCOUNTABILITY AND QUALITY IMPROVEMENT
THROUGH PRACTICE-BASED STUDIES

1960s

Allen RE (1962). A study of subjects discussed by elderly patients in group counseling. *Social Casework*, July.

Berkman B, Rehr H (1966). *A Study of Aging Ward Patients Served*. Monograph. New York: The Mount Sinai Medical Center, June.

Berkman B, Rehr H (1969). *Effects of Differential Timing of Social Service Intervention with the Aged*. Monograph. New York: The Mount Sinai Medical Center.

Rashbaum W, Rehr H, Paneth J, Greenberg M (1963). Pregnancy in unmarried women, medical and social characteristics. *The Mount Sinai Journal of Medicine*, 30(1):33–45.

Ravich R, Rehr H, Goodrich C (1969). Hospital ombudsman smooths flow of services and communication. *Hospitals, 43*:56–61.

Rehr H, Berkman B (1967). Aging ward patients and the hospital social service department. *Journal of the American Geriatrics Society, 15*(12):1153–1162.

Rehr H, Rashbaum W, Paneth J, Greenberg M (1962). *A Study of Extra-Marital Pregnancies at the Mount Sinai Hospital.* Monograph. New York: Departments of Obstetrics and Gynecology, and Social Work Services, The Mount Sinai Medical Center.

Rehr H, Rashbaum W, Paneth J, Greenberg M (1963). Use of Social Services by Unmarried Mothers. *Children, 10*(1):11–16.

Siegel D, Pomrinse D, Rehr H, Berkman B (1968). *Utilization of In-patient Services by the Elderly.* Monograph. New York: The Mount Sinai Medical Center.

Stein F, Siegel D (1966). Survey of tasks and functions of social workers in the health field, its implications and challenges. *Proceedings of the Second Conference for Social Workers in the Health Field. National Conference of Jewish Communical Services.* Washington, DC:(May 14–18):87–92.

1970s

Berkman B, Rehr H (1970). Unanticipated Consequences of the Casefinding System in Hospital Social Service. *Social Work, 15*(2):63–68.

Berkman B (1970). *Social Service Casefinding for the Hospitalized Elderly with Reference to Source of Referral and Timing of Intervention. Dissertation.* New York: Columbia University.

Berkman B, Rehr H, Siegel D, Pomrinse D, Paneth J (1971). Utilization of in-patients services by elderly. *Journal of the American Geriatrics Society, 19*(11):933–946.

Berkman B, Rehr H (1972). The sick role cycle and the timing of social work interventions. *The Social Service Review, 46*(4):567–580.

Berkman B, Rehr H (1973). Early social service casefinding for hospitalized patients: An experiment. *The Social Service Review, 47*(2):256–265.

Berkman B, Rehr H (1973). Social service casefinding in the hospital: Its influence on the utilization of social services. *American Journal of Public Health, 63*(10): 857–862.

Berkman B, Rehr H (1974). The search for early indicators of social service need among elderly hospital patients. *Journal of American Geriatrics Society, XXII*(10): 416–421.

Berkman B, Rehr H (1975). Elderly patients and their families: Factors related to satisfaction with hospital social services. *The Gerontologist, 15*(6):524–528.

Berkman B, Rehr H (1977). Seven steps to audit. *Social Work in Health Care, 2*(3): 295–303.

Berkman B (1977). Are social service audit systems feasible? Experience with a hospital-based and a regional approach. *Development of Professional Standards Review for Hospital Social Work.* Chicago, IL: American Hospital Association: 37–43.

Berkman B, Rehr H (1978). Seven steps in hospital applied social work research. In N Bracht (Ed.). *Social Work in Health Care: A Guide to Professional Practice.* New York: Haworth Press.

Berkman B, Rehr H (1978). Social work undertakes its own audit. *Social Work in Health Care, 3*(3).

Berkman B (1979). Practice-oriented research-principles and methods. In J Morse, M Shipsey (Eds.). Monograph. *Successful Social Living for Sensory Deprived Persons*. Boston, MA:83–87.

Chernesky R, Young AT (1979). Developing a peer review system. In H Rehr (Ed.). *Professional Accountability for Social Work Practice*. New York: Prodist: 74–91.

Lowe JI (1978). Quality assurance in dialysis: The role of the social worker. *Journal of Dialysis*, 2(1):43–53.

Paneth J, Lipsky H (1979). Utilization review and social work's role. In H Rehr (Ed.). *Professional Accountability for Social Work Practice: A Search for Concepts and Guidelines*. New York: Prodist:27–47.

Ravich R, Rehr H (1974). Ombudsman program provides feedback. *Hospitals*, 48(18):63–67.

Rehr H (1975). Models of accountability. In WT Hall, GC St. Denis (Eds.). *Proceedings: Quality Assurance in Social Services in Health Programs for Mothers and Children*. USDHEW. University of Pittsburgh (April):63–66.

Rehr H (1975). Quality and quantity assurance: Issues for social services in health. In WT Hall, GC St. Denis (Eds.). *Proceedings: Quality Assurance in Social Services in Health Programs for Mothers and Children*. USDHEW. University of Pittsburgh (April):35–47.

Rehr H (1977). Quality and quantity assurance: An editorial. *Social Work in Health Care*, 2(2):135–138.

Rehr H (1977). Professional standards review and utilization review: The challenge to social work. Monograph. *Development of Professional Standards Review for Hospital Social Work*. Chicago, IL: American Hospital Association:23–36.

Rehr H, Berkman B (1979). Social needs of the hospitalized elderly: A classification. In A Harbert, L Ginsberg (Eds.). *Human Services for Older Adults: Concepts and Skills*. Belmont, CA: Wadsworth:285–294.

Rehr H (Ed.) (1979). *Professional Accountability for Social Work Practice: A Search for Concepts and Guidelines*. New York: Prodist.

Rehr H (1979). An adventure in professional accountability. In H Rehr (Ed.). *Professional Accountability for Social Work Practice: A Search for Concepts and Guidelines*. New York: Prodist:1–15.

Rehr H (1979). The climate is set for quality assurance: Implications for social work. In H Rehr (Ed.). *Professional Accountability for Social Work Practice: A Search for Concepts and Guidelines*. New York: Prodist:16–26.

Rehr H (1979). Patient care evaluation (audits): Social work prerequisites and current approaches. *Professional Accountability for Social Work Practice: A Search for Concepts and Guidelines*. New York: Prodist:92–110.

Rehr H (1979). Looking to the future. In H Rehr (Ed.). *Professional Accountability for Social Work Practice: A Search for Concepts and Guidelines*. New York:Prodist: 150–168.

Reinherz H, Berkman B, Grob M, Ewalt P (1977). Training in accountability: A social work mandate. *Health and Social Work*, 2(2):43.

Rosenberg G (1976). Data gathering systems in evaluation and research. *National Association of Private Psychiatric Hospitals Journal*, 8(3):31–34.

Rosenberg G (1979). Continuing education and the self-directed worker. In H Rehr (Ed.). *Professional Accountability for Social Work Practice: A Search for Concepts and Guidelines*. New York: Prodist:111–127.

Topper D, Zofnass J, Smith E, Parsons J (1979). The professional staff views accountability. In H Rehr (Ed.). *Professional Accountability for Social Work Practice: A Search for Concepts and Guidelines.* New York: Prodist:142–149.
Young AT (1979). The chart notation. In H Rehr (Ed.). *Professional Accountability for Social Work Practice: A Search for Concepts and Guidelines.* New York: Prodist: 62–73.

1980s

Abramovsky I, Godmilow L, Hirschhorn K, Smith JR (1980). Analysis of a follow-up of genetics counseling. In K Berg, J Book, J Mohr (Eds.). *Clinical Genetics,* 17:1–12.
Bennett C, Grob G (1982). The social worker new to health care: Basic learning tasks. *Social Work in Health Care,* 8(2):49–64.
Bennett C (1984). Testing the value of written information for patients and families in discharge planning. *Social Work in Health Care,* 9(3):95–97.
Berkman B, Rehr H, Rosenberg G (1980). A social work department develops and tests a screening mechanism to identify high social risk situations. *Social Work in Health Care,* 5(4):373–385.
Berkman B (1980). The psychosocial problems and outcome: An external validity study. *Health and Social Work,* 5(3):5 21.
Berkman B, Weissman A (1983). Research: A central component of practice. In R Miller, H Rehr (Eds.). *Social Work Issues in Health Care.* Englewood Cliffs, NJ: Prentice-Hall:221–251.
Bernstein SR (1990). Contracted services: Issues for the non-profit agency manager. *Sector Quality,* 22:429–443.
Berrier J, Sperling R, Preisinger J, Mason J, Walther, V (1991). HIV/AIDS education in a pre-natal clinic: An assessment. *AIDS Education and Prevention,* 3(2):100–117.
Black RB (1989). A 1 and 6 month follow-up of prenatal diagnosis patients who lost pregnancies. *Prenatal Diagnosis,* 9:794–804.
Gantt AB, Goldstein G, Pinsky S (1989). Family understanding of psychiatric illness. *Community Mental Health Journal,* 25(2):101–108.
Kane JM, Rifkin A, Woerner M, Reardon GT, Sarantakos S, Schiebel D, Ramme Lorenzi J (1983). Low dose neuroleptics in the treatment of outpatient schizophrenics. *Archives of General Psychiatry,* 40(8):893–896.
Kane J, Quitkin F, Wegner J, Rosenberg G, Borenstein M (1983). Attitudinal changes of involuntarily committed patients following treatment. *Archives of General Psychiatry,* 40:374–377.
Kirsten L, Rosenberg G, Smith H (1981). Cognitive changes during the menstrual cycle. *International Journal Psychiatry in Medicine,* 10(4):339–346.
Kornfield P, Landman L, Stern D, Gross H, Silberman JM (eds.) (1983). Psychosocial aspects of myasthenia gravis. *Psychosocial Aspects of Muscular Dystrophy and Allied Diseases,* 19:177–182.
Morrison B, Rehr H (1985). Evaluating the consortium: Planners, faculty, preceptors, and graduates. In H Rehr, P Caroff (Eds.). *A New Model in an Academic-practice Partnership.* Lexington, MA: Ginn Press:39–64.
Morrison B, Rehr H, Rosenberg G (1985). How well are you doing? Evaluation strategies for practice. In C Germain (Ed.). *Advances in Clinical Social Work Practice.* Silver Spring, MD: National Association of Social Workers:218–231.

Poliandro E (1989). *Men, Women and Work: A Study of Involvement in Work and Non-work Activities, As Indices for Continued Identity Development in Adulthood*. Dissertation. New York University.

Reardon GT, Blumenfield S, Weissman AL, Rosenberg G (1988). Findings and implications from preadmission screening of elderly patients waiting for elective surgery. *Social Work in Health Care, 13*(3):57–63.

Rehr H, Berkman B, Rosenberg G (1980). Screening for high social risk: Principles and problems. *Social Work, 25*(5):403–406.

Rehr H, Berkman B, Rosenberg G (1980). A new approach to appraising of student field experiences in health settings. In P Caroff, M Mailick (Eds.). *Social Work in Health Services: An Academic-Practice Partnership*. New York: Prodist:131–153.

Rehr H (1982). Trends in social work quality assurance. *Quality Review Bulletin, Special Edition*, Spring:2.

Rehr H, Berkman B (1985). Social service casefinding in the hospital: Its influence on the utilization of social services. *Social Work Practice II: SUNY School of Social Work, Stonybrook*. Lexington, MA: Ginn Press:95–99.

Rehr H, Caroff P, Wilson M (1985). The participants deliberate. In H Rehr, P Caroff (Eds.). *A New Model in an Academic-practice Partnership*. Lexington, MA: Ginn Press:71–79.

Rehr H (1989). Using client satisfaction as an indicator of effectiveness: A brief review. In BS Vourlekis, DC Leukenfeld (Eds.). *Making Our Case*. Silver Spring, MD: National Association of Social Workers.

Rosenberg G, Speedling E, Rehr H, Morrison B (1985). Some effects of a hospital strike on patient satisfaction. *The Mount Sinai Journal of Medicine, 52*(4):259–264.

Rosenberg G, Clarke S (1987). The study: Purpose and method. In G Rosenberg, S Clarke (Eds.). *Social Workers in Health Care Management: The Move to Leadership*. New York: Haworth Press:1–4.

Rosenstein ED, Godmilow L, Hirschhorn K (1980). An assessment of physician knowledge of Tay Sachs disease. *The Mount Sinai Journal of Medicine, 47*(1):1–4.

Shein L (1987). *Social Workers' Perception and Practices in Relation to the Children of Psychiatrically Hospitalized Patients*. Dissertation. New York University.

Showers N (1988). *Factors Associated with Graduate Social Work Student Satisfaction in Hospital Field Education Programs*. Dissertation. City University of New York.

Silberman, JM (1986). *Spouses' Perception of the Impact of Myasthenia Gravis on Marital Interaction*. Dissertation. New York University.

Silverton M (1988). *Assessing Mental Health Problems in Minority Boys*. Dissertation. *Dissertation Abstract International 48*.

Simon EP (1988). Integrating research and practice in the workplace. *Social Work Research and Abstracts*, Summer:4–5.

Siris SG, Rifkin A, Reardon GT (1982). Response of post-psychotic depression to adjunctive imipramine or amitriptyline. *Journal of Clinical Psychiatry, 43*(12): 485–486.

Siris SG, Rifkin A, Reardon GT (1983). Comparative side effects to imipramine, benzotropine or their combination. *Journal of Psychiatry,140*(8):1069–1071.

Speedling E, Morrison B, Rehr H, Rosenberg G (1983). Patient satisfaction: Closing the gap between provider and consumer. *Quality Review Bulletin, 9*(8):224–228.

Young AT (1980). *An Exploratory Study of the Educational Process of Parents of Chronically Ill Children: Diabetes and Asthma*. Dissertation. Columbia University Teachers' College.

1990s

Bernstein SR (1991). Contracted services: Issues for the non-profit agency manager. *Sector Quality, 22:*429–443.

Berrier J, Sperling R, Preisinger J, Mason J, Walther V (1991). HIV/AIDS education in a prenatal clinic: An assessment. *AIDS Education and Prevention, 3*(2):100–117.

Black RB (1991). Women's voices after pregnancy loss: couples' patterns of communication and support. *Social Work in Health Care, 16*(2):19–36.

Gantt A, Pinsky S, Rock B, Rosenberg E (1990). Practice and research: An integrative approach. *Journal of Teaching in Social Work, 4*(1):129–143.

Gantt A, Pinsky S (1990). Practice research center: A field/class model to teach research, practice and values. In D Schneck (Ed.). *Field Education in Social Work.* Dubuque, IA: Kendall-Hunt.

Gantt A, Levine J (1990). The roles of social work in psycho-biological research. *Social Work in Health Care, 15*(2):63–75.

Holden G, Moncher MS (1990). Self-efficacy of children, and adolescents: A meta-analysis. *Psychological Reports, 66*(June):1044–1046.

Holden G, Barker KM (1990). Potential for technological dependency: An example. *Social Work Research and Abstracts, 26:*35–36.

Holden G, Rosenberg G (1991). Editorial: Research challenges for social workers in health. *Social Work in Health Care, 16*(2):1–4.

Holden G (1991). *The Relationship of Self-Efficacy Appraisals to Subsequent Self-related Outcomes: A Meta-analysis.* Dissertation. Columbia University. October. Also in *Social Work in Health Care* (1991), *16*(1):53–94.

Katch M (1990). *Select Worker Attributes and Their Relationship to Initiation of Group in Health Care Setting (Group Training).* Dissertation. New York University.

Moncher MS, Holden G, Trimble JE (1990). Substance abuse among Native American youth. *Journal of Consulting and Clinical Psychology, 58*(4):418–415.

Moncher MS, Holden G, Schinke SP (1991). Psychosocial correlates of adolescent substance abuse: A review of current etiological constructs. *International Journal of the Addictions, 26:*377–414.

Razin A, O'Dowd MA, Nathan A, Rodriguez I, Goldfield A, Martin C, Goulet L, Shefter S, Mezun P, Mosca J (1991). Suicidal behavior among inner-city Hispanic adolescent females. *General Hospital Psychiatry, 13:*45–58.

Rehr H (1990). Discharge planning: an ongoing function of quality care. *Quality Review Bulletin, 12*(2):47–50.

Rehr H (1991). Quality assurance and leadership enhancement. In C Irizarry, C James (Eds.). *Achieving Excellence in Health Social Work.* Adelaide, Australia: Flinders Press: 26–53.

Rehr H (1991). Integrating practice and research. In C Irizarry, C James (Eds.). *Achieving Excellence in Health Social Work.* Adelaide Australia: Flinders Press: 54–84.

Rehr H (1991). High social risk screening. In C Irizarry, C James (Eds.). *Achieving Excellence in Health Social Work.* Adelaide, Australia: Flinders Press:97–126.

Simon EP (1991, May). Research for the research phobic: developing research expertise in hospital social work. *Health and Social Work, 16*(2):118–122.

Weiss HM, Simon R, Levi J, Foster A, Hubbard M, Aledorf L (1991). Compliance in a comprehensive hemophilia center and its implication for home care. *Family Systems Medicine, 9*(2):112–120.

6

Discharge Planning: A Key Function

Susan Blumenfield, Claire Bennett, and Helen Rehr

Discharge planning plays a major role in securing a continuum of care for patients that is in harmony with their biopsychosocial needs. The American Hospital Association (AHA) defines discharge planning as "any activity or set of activities that facilitates the transition of the patient from one environment to another" (Rossen, 1985; p. 2). AHA's protocol describes the complexity of discharge planning on four levels of outcome:

1. patient and family understanding of patient diagnosis, anticipated level of functioning, and the need for medical follow-up;
2. specialized training and instruction to ensure good posthospital care;
3. coordination of community supports; and/or
4. relocation of the patient through the coordination of support systems to another health care facility.

This description underscores the roles and expertise of many health care providers within the institution and the community. Implementing discharge planning activities, and their coordination, are central functions of the hospital-based social worker. Today's social workers monitor comprehensive discharge planning services in a case management context. The case management approach to discharge planning requires several professional skills, including the ability to assess risk factors in aftercare, enhance the informal support of the family, and access the formal support of community resources as needed. Case management calls for rapid incorporation of the assessment into a plan of action, and current knowledge of entitlement and program resources. The discharge process requires interpersonal skills to form working relationships with patients, families, and providers and achieve optimal planning that supports patients in their own or a planned environment.

THE CHALLENGE

The evolution and status of discharge planning as a professional social work function follow the broader course of social work professional development throughout the 20th century, reflecting changes in practice and theory and their effect on values and attitudes within the field. Social workers have been invested in a discharge planning role with patients since 1906 when Dr. Richard Cabot identified the need to learn the personal and environmental factors that would affect a discharged patient's ability to deal with medical recommendations and achieve health gains (Cannon, 1913).

In 1915 Flexner denied social work professional status, seeing it primarily as a "mediating force" lacking a central core of knowledge. In an effort to ensure professional status as treatment experts and create a theoretical core of knowledge, social workers turned to existing psychological (primarily psychoanalytic) theories, closely following the medical model of diagnosis and treatment. As they sought greater professionalism, a disquietude about discharge planning began to surface. From an intellectual viewpoint, discharge planning increasingly was viewed as a routine, administrative task and was often delegated to paraprofessionals. "Diminished was the response to environmental problems and their impact on people that had characterized the efforts of the forerunners of professional social workers" (Davidson, 1978; p. 46).

From the mid-1920s to the 1960s, although social workers continued to handle the discharge function, they accorded it low status. Definitions of discharge planning ran in many directions. "Is it a complex process calling for sophisticated skills or a simple one requiring merely the ability to follow protocols?" (James, 1985). Although hospital administrators argued that institutional responsibilities to patients began and ended at the hospital door, they also demanded that social work departments coordinate and implement the discharge planning function for the institution.

Resistance to giving discharge planning a primary role dissolved in 1966 when Medicare and Medicaid programs were established. Medicare legislation transformed hospital discharge planning into a government-mandated activity that required master's-prepared social workers to provide services to inpatient Medicare and Medicaid patients and handicapped children. All insurances followed with an accredited reimbursement for inpatient social services.

Hospital construction and admissions expanded rapidly in this period, as did technological advances, all of which often resulted in fragmented, episodic, and depersonalized care. National fiscal crises in the 1970s and 1980s resulted in cutbacks in services and ultimately in the introduction of Diagnosis Related Groups (DRGs), which curtailed the past luxury of open-ended hospital stays. Discharge planning became a central concern to social policy planners and to hospital and social work administrators. Sound discharge planning, including aftercare planning, became vital not only to the financial survival of institutions, but to their image as caring, efficient, and responsible players in the health care market. With their emphasis on the individual and the place of the family and significant others in patient support, their knowledge of community resources, and their collaborative relationship with other primary health care providers, social workers reclaimed the domain. They recognized that quality discharge required the most sophisticated skills to influence attitudes and behaviors and to safeguard sound aftercare for clients.

Commenting on social work's response to DRGs and the cost-containment measures of the 1980s, Carlton (1989) said "discharge planning is an example of another role in which health social workers should take pride in their ability to respond rapidly and flexibly to dramatic, often unanticipated change without losing sight of the profession's purpose and values. In response to DRG mandates, social workers gained a deepened understanding of the nature of short-term intervention and skill in delivering services on this basis; the implications [of this discovery] go beyond the discharge role" (p. 229).

In parallel developments, profound changes were occurring in theory and practice within the behavioral and social sciences, psychiatry, psychology, and social work itself. In the physical sciences, the linear or Newtonian model of cause and effect was supplanted by the general systems theory which focused on patterns and on the processes and flows of energy and information. Among system elements a shift from certainties to probabilities occurred. Social work favored the systematic perspective of ecology or that of the life sciences, which emphasized the degree of fit between people's rights, needs, capacities, and goals on the one hand and the quality of the social and physical environment on the other (Germain & Gitterman, 1987). Through the major influences of crisis intervention, short-term treatment models, and stress, coping, and adaptation theories, the fields of psychiatry and psychology further validated social work discharge activities. These activities centered on helping patients and families cope with and adapt to illness. As a result of these emphases, the "clinical" nature of discharge planning received new attention in practice and professional literature.

THE RELEVANT LITERATURE

Publications confirm the principle that discharge planning is a concept/ function that requires periodic redefinition, as medical care, technology, funding sources, support networking, patient and family attitudes, and behaviors and resources change. Despite changes, fundamental skills and practice concepts remain in place. They can be classified along five domains: continuity of care, high social-risk screening, ethical dilemmas, program planning, and practice skills.

CONTINUITY OF CARE

Forty years ago, publications about polio victims discharged home focused on the need for continuous care to achieve enhanced physical and social functioning. Discharge plans centered on the patient's sense of "body image" and his "at-home" network of support in a physical-spatial as well as psychological and social sense. Linkage between the medical institution and a home care agency ensured continuity of care. This reciprocity of service initiated an early type of case management approach.

In 1988, social work leaders offered a more current perspective of an expanded and redefined discharge planning process—social health care management. In this process, illness is viewed on a continuum in which the social work role extends to primary and secondary prevention as well as to the traditional tertiary or acute-care phase, thus maintaining the patient-family connection to the medical center for pre- and posthospital social-health care and medical treatment. While recognizing the major impact of acute hospitalization, social-health care management is also concerned with the patient's situation before and after the acute event, thus revealing possibilities for creative program planning and social work intervention. Such programs, in which hospital and community resources are combined to meet the biopsychosocial needs of patients along a continuum of care, might include:

- hospital-based consultation services for attending physicians in a fee-for-service model under the direction of the social service department;
- social work services based in physicians' private offices;
- psychosocial service in the emergency service;
- preadmission social work screening and consultation;
- hospital-based case-management services for the elderly and disabled in which social workers offer entitlement information and monitor service delivery within the hospital and community;

- health education and health promotion (wellness) programs for patients and community members;
- post-discharge follow-up services that include evaluation of discharge services and patient satisfaction. This program is marketable to institutions in that it measures patient satisfaction and reduces the need for rehospitalization; and
- interim home care programs that offer personal care for a limited time as a stop-gap while arranging for longer-term needs.

Social-health care management is a proactive strategy of discharge planning that not only provides patients and families with a comprehensive plan of psychosocial health care but also uses hospital and community resources in a structured, cost-efficient, and productive way compatible with the present health care environment.

High Social-Risk Screening

To offer quality discharge planning, it is essential that those in need of comprehensive services be identified early in their hospitalization. In the mid-1960s, as social workers studied who used the institution, they uncovered selectivity biases among other health care providers regarding whom they referred to social services, and when—referrals occurred on the day before or day of discharge, impeding the ability to plan effectively. Further exploration revealed that the traditional referral system left social workers totally dependent on others; social work had relinquished the right to set its own priorities and thus patients and families were deprived sound aftercare planning. High social-risk screening was developed and social work began to screen at preadmission, admission, and no later than 24 hours after admission. Although telephone prescreening of elective admissions did not shorten stays, patients responded positively.

High social-risk screening by social workers was institutionalized in hospitals across the country and became an indicator of access to social services and a quality assurance measure, enabling social workers to ascertain who was at high social-risk, triaging patients simultaneously. The variables that surfaced most frequently in identifying those at-risk included:

- age greater than 80 or greater than 70 with disability;
- living alone or without residence;
- multiple illnesses;
- limited social functioning, physical functioning, and ability to perform selected activities of daily living;

- depression, confusion, and slow comprehension;
- incontinence;
- repeated admission in the past six months;
- lack of a readily available social support network; and
- limited financial resources.

By and large, any combination of two or more of these factors justified an assessment for high social-risk. Social work gained professional status in claiming its own casefinding mechanisms and drew on its skills early to offer quality care to patients and families. As social work continued to study the outcomes for discharged patients, it uncovered the many problems that they and their families encountered.

ETHICAL DILEMMAS

Discharge planning addresses the patient's right to receive basic services that will permit transfer from the institution to home or a suitable alternate environment. The rights to information about illness, resources, and options are basic to sound decision making. Personal, culturally based values often affect the decision-making process, and communication problems in the complex hospital environment obscure decisions and issues of self-determination. Experiences reflect that conflicts between internal and external staff require constant deliberation for resolution.

PROGRAM PLANNING

The process and rationale for program development are closely allied to discharge planning. A legal clinic, for example, was established on the basis that discharge planning social workers had to be informed about the complicated legal structures related to change of assets and rulings on competence and guardianship, to name but a few. Medicaid and Medicare regulations also require frequent educational updates. The legal strictures required application on a case-by-case basis. The open forum in which workers exchange problems and planning with a legal expert has become an invaluable teaching tool for practitioners.

An interim home care program developed with a community home care agency illustrated the advantages of offering comprehensive support early to a group of at-risk patients who might otherwise require protracted hospital stays. For a selected number of patients at-risk for a long stay, the program allowed early and safe discharge by drawing on available and relevant community resources. At-risk patients given comprehensive support and care in their homes benefitted from an early return to their familiar surroundings. Patients and family members preferred the early discharge to a protracted hospital stay.

PRACTICE SKILLS

Many of the practice issues in discharge planning are relevant to clinical interventions and social work roles and functions and include the use of empathy and information to establish a client-worker relationship. One author addressed social workers' attempts to secure early entry into high-risk situations by introducing an informational pamphlet about certain illnesses. Social workers hoped the pamphlets would promote health education; later study revealed that although the experiment did not achieve an educational objective, the pamphlets promoted easy social worker access to patients, facilitated "making a case" between worker and client, and proved successful as a tool to establish the relationship.

In other instances, the complexities of the institution resulted in fragmentation of care. For example, patients discharged from the institution and referred for outpatient care would arrive on the appointed day to find their clinic doctor did not have their chart record. A revised discharge form containing essential medical information was developed and provided to patients at discharge to give the clinic physician. The new procedure was successful and ensured ongoing knowledgeable care.

CONCLUSION

Hospitalized patients have highly individualized needs. Each discharge requires a plan that safeguards care at home. The discharge planning function is complex and requires multiple skills. In general, it requires psychological knowledge, a biopsychosocial approach to care, which involves a range of health care professionals in a shared relationship, and a network of community-based services.

Discharge planning, as a concept and a function, cannot be limited to medical oversight, but must be redefined in a social-health case-management context. Any health care reform planning must encompass safeguarding access to and coordination of care, comprehensiveness and continuity of care, development of health promotional programs, and availability of aftercare. If those in need could be found before illness strikes, primary prevention would serve. For those suffering from ongoing chronic illnesses and disabilities, a continuum of care is needed before, during, and after hospitalization.

Social workers validated their availability to doctors in offices, in emergency rooms, in preadmission consultation, and no later than at-admission screening. They demonstrated that social workers can hold key roles in health education and health promotion programs. Their continued roles and functions within the institution remain critical. The posthospital role for social work calls for systematic follow-up and monitoring of medical and social work services.

Social workers' broad knowledge of the client-provider community systems makes them prime coordinators of care, or case managers, in today's parlance. Social workers today spend as much time with patients and families in counseling and social services as do physicians in medical care. Studies of consumer satisfaction with social work services in discharge planning reflect positive opinion.

It is ironic that discharge planning as an area of social work expertise is vulnerable yet again to forces of negative pressure, not within the profession but within the political arena of conservative deprofessionalism and fiscal downsizing in health care. As with many social welfare programs, one can but hope that the strength of consumerism and the value put on a caring and responsible society will prevail. In the meantime, social work continues to be the primary provider for discharge services, but the obligation for staff to review experiences and project new programs, interventions, and practice insights into the discharge planning process is critical, as the populace faces new health care delivery systems, particularly managed care. It suggests that discharge planning is more than discharge, but a comprehensive continuum of care that relates to preadmission and postdischarge, based on the individual's biopsychosocial needs. The new programs, many developed by industry, insurers, and providers, require social workers to articulate these insights in a variety of forums, including publishing.

MOUNT SINAI REFERENCES

Discharge Planning: A Key Function

1970s

Berkman B, Rehr H (1970). Unanticipated consequences of the casefinding system in hospital social service. *Social Work, 15*(2):63–68.
Wagner D, Cohen MC (1978). Social workers, class and professionalism. *Catalyst, 1*.

1980s

Bennett C, Beckerman N (1986). The drama of discharge: Worker/supervisor perspectives. *Social Work in Health Care, 11*(3):1–12.

Blumenfield S (1986). Editorial: Discharge planning: Changes for hospital social work in a new health care climate. *Quality Review Bulletin, 12*(2):51–54.

Blumenfield S, Lowe JI (1987). Data, values and decision making: A template for analyzing ethical dilemmas in discharge planning. *Health and Social Work, 12*(1):47–56.

Blumenfield S, Rosenberg G (1988). Toward a network of social health services: Redefining discharge planning and expanding the social work domain. *Social Work in Health Care, 13*(4):31–48.

Ravich R, Weissman GK (1981). Revised discharge form improves continuity of care. *The Hospital Medical Staff, 10*(2):12–19.

Rehr H (1984). Commentary: Discharge planning. *Quality Review Bulletin, 10*(12):546–547.

Rehr H (1986). Discharge planning: An ongoing function of quality care. *Quality Review Bulletin, 12*(2):47–50.

Young AT (1987). Discharge planning and ethical dilemmas. *Discharge Planning Update, 7*:(July/August):3–4.

1990s

Dobrof J (1991). DRGs and the social worker's role in discharge planning. *Social Work in Health Care, 16*(2):37–54.

Rehr H (1990). Discharge planning: An ongoing function of quality care. *Examples of Monitoring and Evaluation in Hospital Social Work Services and Discharge Planning*. Monograph. Chicago, IL: Joint Commission for the Accreditation of Healthcare Organizations.

Schwartz P, Blumenfield S, Simon EP (1990). The interim homecare program: An innovative discharge planning alternative. *Health and Social Work, 15*(2):152–160.

Simon EP (1991). Interim home care meets both patients' and hospital needs. *Picker/Commonwealth Report,1,* (Spring):7–8.

7

Collaboration and Consultation: Key Social Work Roles in Health Care

Helen Rehr, Susan Blumenfield, and Gary Rosenberg

Two concepts shape the philosophy that health care must be comprehensive, coordinated, and continuous:

- the introduction of a biopsychosocial focus to medical care,
- [which resulted in] the recognition that medical service required a social-health model.

These concepts developed from recognition of the important relationship between psychological and social-environmental factors in sickness and disability and their significance in maintaining optimum living patterns and health. A biopsychosocial diagnosis is a requirement in a social-health care model. Although many patients simply require the interventions of their solo-practitioner physicians, those with chronic or severe illness, multiple disorders, and social disorders almost routinely require consultation or collaboration among health care providers to manage complex biopsychosocial needs.

From its early beginnings, the social work profession sought the medical profession's recognition of psychosocial components in medical care and social work's contributions to the comprehensive care of patients and families. In the early history of social work services, social workers followed physicians' directions. When physicians were concerned about an individual's compliance and/or deprivations in the environment and lack of community resources to support medical recommendations, they turned to social workers. Although social workers sometimes were referred to as doctors' "handmaidens," the birth of medical social work resulted from both professions' recognition of the need to address the social and psychological problems related to sickness.

As medicine advanced its knowledge and technology and conquered many of the infectious diseases, it began to face new disorders that arose from environmental problems and from individuals' social and behavioral patterns. And as medicine recognized that disease and disability contained biopsychosocial phenomena, and social workers (and others) introduced the content into patient care, the shift to a social-health care model began, but not without struggle. Social workers strived to develop and maintain collaborative relationships with the medical and health professions; they wrote frequently about the success of programs developed collaboratively, and their challenges. It is social workers who bring an understanding of patient and family psychosocial situations to medical discussion.

DEFINITIONS

Consultation puts relevant knowledge and skills at the disposal of others for their use on behalf of the client, the service and/or the institution. Consultation can occur among members of the same profession or between professions and disciplines. It generally is episodic. The consultant does not initiate the request, and is not responsible for how his client uses the consultation. The consultee chooses the consultant for the consultant's knowledge, seeking additional information to enhance his professional commitment to the client or to the situation. The consultee poses the questions he or she wants the consultant to address, and is at liberty to use the information or not. The client or relevant others may be involved in the consultation.

Collaboration is a complex and dynamic process. It occurs when two or more providers cooperate and/or assist in providing social-health care either directly or indirectly with individuals and/or families, or, in a broader context, in programs or policy formulation. A wide range of modalities exist in which collaboration can occur—a team of providers, a partnership in care between two professionals of different orientation, consultation, inter- or multiprofessional practice or educational endeavors, and a milieu focus are but a few. The effectiveness of social workers in health care settings is governed by their ability to work collaboratively. Whether employed in a dyadic relationship or in teamwork, collaboration requires a high degree of cooperation to be successful. Each participant must believe that she has something to contribute and that the contribution will be recognized in overall decision making and planning.

These expectations are not without their difficulties. Different professions bring different values, attitudes, and skills to deliberations. Even projected goals can be different. Although objectives need not be alike, the interactive process in the working relationship is critical. Dialogue should create shared understanding and cooperation among participants in the collaborative process.

Social workers' counseling skills are essential to the collaborative process. Each member of the team must first manage her sense of autonomy and address any competitive feelings. Each professional must become aware of the professional culture and language of team members and recognize the unique knowledge and skills, along with commitment to quality care that each brings to the process. Interdependence must occur.

THE CHALLENGE

Despite greater acceptance of biopsychosocial factors in health care, the social-health mission of institutions, and physician education in the biopsychosocial etiology of disease, sound collaboration does not come easily but it is often caught in organizational and discipline constraints. The governance of rights as well as the prerogatives of nonphysician personnel in social-health settings and the continued acceptance of physician dominance in decision making are powerful factors that influence collaboration. Training members of each health discipline about integrated dimensions in social-health care and applying integration to team practice are essential.

The relationship between the consumer and providers in interaction is the most critical factor in achieving mutually desired outcomes. It also is the most vulnerable. Providers must be as sensitive to this relationship in collaboration as they are to that among the different health disciplines.

THE RELEVANT LITERATURE

Social workers have been conscious of the constant need to remind physicians, other health care providers, the institution, and reimbursing agencies about the benefits of social services to patients. Their publications reflect growth in collaborative efforts and note the problems and conflicts that have occurred as well as the changing relationships among the different disciplines.

CONSULTANTS TO PHYSICIANS

As early as 1953, social work identified its role as consultants to physicians in providing a broader dimension to medical care. In bringing a biopsychosocial focus to the diagnosis and treatment of patients' ailments, social work identified a set of guidelines and the skills needed to reach physicians. When the poliomyelitis epidemic occurred, it became clear that physicians needed knowledge of the social components of an illness. Social work demonstrated that social, vocational, and environmental rehabilitation were as important to patient recovery as physical rehabilitation. Health professionals recognized the interdependence of these components as essential to optimum rehabilitation.

Physicians and social workers each demonstrated the concept of patient self-image in body awareness, and physicians gave their social work colleagues the role of helping patients to regain self-worth and become motivated to regain quality of life along with whatever physical restoration could be achieved. This early collaboration between medicine and social work was brought forward and applied to the care of patients with other major chronic disorders, including coronary disabilities, hemophilia, myasthenia gravis, genetic diseases, and the cancers, to name a few.

COMMUNITY AGENCY INTERRELATIONSHIPS

The work of the late 1950s illustrated the need for community agency interrelationships within the medical institution to ensure a continuum of care. Collaborative networking supported the needs of the polio victims as they returned home. Later, when discharged Medicaid patients required ongoing 'at-home' services, the interagency network continued. A casefinding health team went to local schools to help children with health problems. Health education teams went into the community to offer preventive services for the elderly, and direct care to children in whom they discovered eye problems. In the 1980s a direct liaison between the institution and community agencies was created and continues today to address the health care needs of local-area residents. To raise awareness of the need for social-health policy and legislation, a staff social worker testified before a congressional subcommittee with her physician colleague about the needs of the hemophiliac patient and family.

INTERPROFESSIONAL CHALLENGES

Social work publications voiced the problems workers encountered with other health care providers, simultaneously identifying key areas in which collaboration had been successful. A few wrote of turf conflicts, role confusion, and the need to put definition to the roles and responsibilities of each of the health care professionals. Others wrote about the support for the interprofessional team approach.

In the early 1960s, as gaps in obstetrical services to unmarried mothers, particularly pregnant teenagers, were demonstrated, a multidisciplinary team was developed to offer guidance in sexual health maintenance and to support stability in interpersonal relationships. Networking developed to promote collaboration and consultation with community organizations. Co-leaders conducted group treatment programs. The concept is now commonplace as social workers, physicians, nurses, and other health care personnel co-lead groups. Health care team members engaged in joint studies of drug abuse, AIDS, psychiatric problems, geriatric issues, breast cancer, and other severe illnesses and disabilities. As social workers, nurses, and doctors worked together, their different professional and personal values became evident. Ethical dilemmas in patient care surfaced frequently and were addressed in open discussion in team meetings and the legal clinic. Cultural diversity was recognized as an important factor in securing compliance in patient management.

DISCHARGE PLANNING

Discharge planning is another major arena in which the integration of biological, psychological, and social factors was seen as critical in postoperative care. A revised discharge form ensures continuity of patient care. Problem-oriented records offer a comprehensive view of individual patients and help providers contribute to more informed joint planning (see also chapter 6).

INTERPROFESSIONAL EDUCATION

Collaboration was expanded to include interprofessional education. The community emphasis in health care in the new medical school offered opportunities for interprofessional education, particularly for medical and social work students. Social work redefined its relationship to academic social work in health care as the social work and medicine connection was refined in service, in medical education, in research, and in program planning and design. A new model in an academic-practice partnership was developed in which a program was designed to include multiple field instructors, multiple institutions, and a medical and social work faculty. The endeavor addressed the prevailing perception of the separateness of social practice and academia and the perceived gap in education for competent entry-level social workers in health care. A consortium comprised of field and school social workers and supported by the institutions, the faculty and administration of the school, and the hospital, enhanced both practice and academic education and has become a model for quality social work-educational collaboration.

CONCLUSION

Achieving quality collaboration, whether on behalf of and with clients or on behalf of social-health programs and policies, is desirable and fraught with obstacles and deterrents. To serve those in need in a social-health context, a biopsychosocial model of care is most effective.

Although biopsychosocial care often is the purview of a single health care provider, it is more comprehensive when provided through multi-professional collaboration; each professional brings unique expertise to creating an integrated diagnostic and treatment focus. "The time is ripe for alliance and coalition building across disciplines. As the health care system moves toward greater emphasis on care in ambulatory settings, ongoing rather than episodic collaboration may become the norm. Success in developing collaborative practice requires that all team members understand common barriers and the strategies needed to minimize them. Social workers can assume leadership in shaping, rather than merely responding to, changing conditions and in the process can contribute to the development of new and more effective models of interdisciplinary patient care" (Abramson & Mizrahi, 1996; p. 280).

MOUNT SINAI REFERENCES

COLLABORATION AND CONSULTATION

1950s

Rehr H (1957). Developing Casework Understanding with a Lay Committee. *Social Work*, 2(3):62–69.
Siegel D (1953). The function of consultation. *Symposium Proceedings, School of Social Work, University of Pittsburgh*. Pittsburgh, PA: School of Social Work, University of Pittsburgh:181–198.

1960s

Dana B, Sheps C (1968). Trends and issues in interprofessional education: Pride, prejudice and progress. *Education for Social Work*, Fall:35–41.

Rehr H, Rashbaum W, Paneth J, Greenberg M (1962). *A Study of Extra-marital Pregnancies at the Mount Sinai Hospital*. Monograph. Departments of Obstetrics and Gynecology, and Social Work Services, The Mount Sinai Hospital.

Rehr H, Rashbaum W, Paneth J, Greenberg M (1963). Use of Social Services by Unmarried Mothers. *Children, 10*(1):11–16.

Schonholz D, Gusberg SB, Astrachan JM, Young AT, Gouley C (1969). An adolescent guidance program: Study in education for marital health. *Obstetrics and Gynecology, 34*(4):611–614.

Sweet A, White E (1961). Social and functional rehabilitation of patients with severe poliomyelitis. *The Mount Sinai Journal of Medicine,* 28:366–280.

White E (1961). The body-image concept in rehabilitating severely handicapped patients. *Social Work, 6*(3):51–58.

1970s

Aufses A, Dana B (1972). Introduction to medicine: A development history and analysis of an interdepartmental course. In VW Lippard, E Purcell (Eds.). *The Changing Medical Curriculum—Report of a Macy Conference*. New York: Josiah Macy, JR FDN.

Bosch S, Merino R, Daniels M, Fischer E, Rosenthal M (1979). A proposed network to improve access to high-quality health care for medicaid-eligible families. *Journal of Community Health, 4*(4):302–311.

Caroff P, Wilson M (1979). Social work education for professional accountability: The Hunter College School of Social Work and Mount Sinai School of Medicine Consortium. In H Rehr (Ed.). *Professional Accountability for Social Work Practice: A Search for Concepts and Guidelines*. New York: Prodist:128–141.

Dana B, Banta HD, Deuschle K (1974). An agenda for the future of interprofessionalism. In H Rehr (Ed.). *Medicine and Social Work: An Exploration in Interprofessionalism*. New York: Prodist:77–88.

Dana B (1977). Consumer health education. *Proceedings of the Academy of Political Science,* 32:182–192.

Dana B (1978). Value dilemmas in the delivery of social health services: Caring, coping and curing. In H Rehr (Ed.). *Ethical Dilemmas in Health Care: A Professional Search for Solutions*. New York: Prodist:25–32.

Daniels M, Bosch SJ (1978). School health planning: A case for interagency collaboration. *Social Work in Health Care, 3*(4):457–467.

Deuschle K, Bosch S, Banta HD, Dana B (1972). The community medicine clerkship: A learner-centered program. *Journal of Medical Education,* 47:931–938.

Gusberg SB, Marinoff S, Hilsen J, Cox L, Young AT, Cameron O (1975). Therapeutic listening: An adolescent guidance program in motivation for contraception. *The Mount Sinai Journal of Medicine, 42*(5):439–444.

Lowe JI, Herranen M (1978). Conflict in teamwork: Understanding roles and relationships. *Social Work in Health Care, 3*(3):323–330.

Mulvihill M, Dana B (1974). The health team in community medicine. In A Amesan (Ed.). *Community Medicine in Developing Countries*. New York: Springer: 423–430.

Paneth J (1972). Social health advocacy program. *American Journal of Public Health,* January:60–63.

Regensburg J (1979). *Toward Education for Health Professions*. New York: Harper & Row.

Regensburg J (1974). A venture in interprofessionalism. In H Rehr (Ed.). *Medicine and Social Work: An Exploration in Interprofessionalism*. New York: Prodist: 35–73.

Rehr H (1970). *Comparison of Health Care Professions on Predicted Outlook of Patient Compliance, and in General Attitudes Regarding Collaboration and Health Care*. Dissertation. Columbia University School of Social Work.

Rehr H (1974). *Medicine and Social Work: An Exploration in Interprofessionalism*. New York: Prodist.

Rehr H (Ed.) (1978). *Ethical Dilemmas in Health Care: A Professional Search for Solutions*. New York: Prodist.

Rehr H, Bosch S (1978). A professional search into values and ethics in health care delivery. In H Rehr (Ed.). *Ethical Dilemmas in Health Care: A Professional Search for Solutions*. New York: Prodist:35–62.

Wincott E (1977). Psychosocial aspects of hemophilia: Problems, prevention, treatment, research, and future directions. *The Mount Sinai Journal of Medicine*, 44(3):438–455.

1980s

Anvaripour PL, Bernard L, Bronter D, Eden A, Kaplan M, Morris J, Ravich R, Schwartz P (1989). Communicating with hearing impaired patients who utilize the services of a major medical center. *The Journal of the Society of Otorhinolaryngology Head and Neck Surgery*, 7(1):24–26.

Blumenfield S (1983). A summer fellowship program in gerontological social work in health care. *Journal of Gerontological Social Work*, 5(3):2–75.

Blumenfield S, Morris J, Sherman FT (1982). The geriatric team in the acute care hospital: An educational and consultation modality. *Journal of the American Geriatrics Society*, 30(10):660–664.

Bosch S, Merino R, Rose D, Julius N (1986). Community participation in New York City: Success or failure? *American Journal of Preventive Medicine*, 2(4):198–204.

Butler RN, Lewis M (1983). Sexual frustration of older women: A brief guide to office counseling. *Medical Aspects of Human Sexuality*, 17(4):65–69.

Butler RN, Lewis M (1986). *Aging and Mental Health: Positive Psychosocial and Biomedical Approaches*. New York: C.V. Mosby. Revised edition, 1991.

Chan JM, Cincotta N (1981). Training students to work with terminally ill children in a child life program. In R Debellis (Ed.). *The Housestaff and Thanatology*. Salem, NH: Arno Press:111–117.

Clarke S, Neuwirth L, Bernstein R (1986). An expanded social work role in a university hospital-based group practice: Service provider, physician educator and organizational consultant. *Social Work in Health Care*, 11(4):1–18.

Dana B (1983). The collaborative process. In R Miller, H Rehr (Eds.). *Social Work Issues in Health Care*. Englewood Cliffs, NJ: Prentice Hall:181–220.

Dana B (1983). The social work-community medicine connection. In G Rosenberg, H Rehr (Eds.). *Advancing Social Work Practice in the Health Care Field*. New York: Haworth Press:11–23.

Elster S, Dobrof R, Rehr H (1981). Synthesis: Geriatrics and gerontology. *Mount Sinai Journal of Medicine*, 48(6):575–577.

Jacobs P, Lurie A, Cuzzi L (1983). Coordination of services to methadone mothers and their addicted newborns. *Health and Social Work*, 8(4):290–298.

Kane J, Quitkin F, Wegner J, Rosenberg G, Borenstein M (1983). Attitudinal changes of involuntarily committed patients following treatment. *Archives of General Psychiatry, 40*:374–377.

Kane JM, Rifkin A, Woerner M, Reardon GT, Sarantakos S, Schieber D, Ramme Lorenzi J (1983). Low dose neuroleptics in the treatment of outpatient schizophrenics. *Archives of General Psychiatry,40*:893–896.

Kirsten L, Rosenberg G, Smith H (1981). Cognitive changes during the menstrual cycle. *International Journal of Psychiatry in Medicine, 10*(4):339–346.

Levy LP (1982). The integration of the foster grandparent program with an acute care psychiatric service. *Social Work in Health Care 8*(1):27–35.

Levy LP, Joyce P, List J (1987). Reconciliations with parents as a treatment goal for adolescents in an acute care psychiatric hospital. *Social Work in Health Care, 13*(1):1–21.

Lewis M (1989). Sexual problems in the elderly, II: Men's vs. women's. Geriatric panel discussion. *Geriatrics, 44*(3):75–86.

Lowe JI, Herranen M (1981). Understanding teamwork: Another look at the concepts. *Social Work in Health Care, 7*:1–11.

Mailick MD, Ashley AA (1981). Politics of interprofessional collaboration: Challenge to advocacy. *Social Casework, 62*(3):131–137.

Mailick MD, Jordan P (1989). A Multi-model approach to collaborative practice. In K Davidson, S Clarke (Eds.). *Social Work in Health Care*. New York: Haworth Press.

Masser I, Caroscio J, *et al.* (1983). The team approach to the care of patients with amyotrophic lateral sclerosis. In LI Charash, SG Wolf (Eds.). *Psychosocial Aspects of Muscular Dystrophy and Allied Diseases*. Springfield, IL: CC Thomas: 159–166.

Nestlebaum A, Siris SG, Rifkin A, Klar H, Reardon GT (1986). *American Journal of Psychiatry, 143*:1170–1171.

Ravich R, Weissman GK (1981). Revised discharge form improves continuity of care. *The Hospital Medical Staff, 10*(2):12–19.

Reardon GT, Rifkin A (1989). The changing pattern of neuroleptic doses over the past decade. *American Journal of Psychiatry,146*:726–729.

Rehr H, Elster S (Eds.) (1981). Geriatrics and gerontology: A multi-disciplinary approach to medical and social problems. *Mount Sinai Journal of Medicine, 48*(6):478, 575–577.

Rifkin A, Reardon GT (1985). Trimipramine in physical illness with depression. *Journal of Clinical Psychiatry, 46*:4–8.

Rifkin A, Wortman R, Reardon GT, Siris SG (1986). Psychotropic medication in adolescents: A review. *Journal of Clinical Psychiatry, 47*:400–408.

Rubenstein S, Wilson M (1982). Collaboration in a hospital: The case of the dying woman. In G Getzel (Ed.). *Gerontological Social Work in Long Term Care*. New York: Haworth Press:169–178.

Siegel ME (1987). Psychosocial aspects of chemotherapy in cancer care: The patient, family and staff. In R Debellis, G Hyman, Seeland I, Kutscher A, Torres C, Barrett V, Siegel ME (Eds.). New York: Haworth Press.

Siris SG, Rifkin A, Reardon GT 1983). Comparative side effects to imipramine, benzotropine or their combination. *Journal of Psychiatry,140*(8):1069–1071.

Siris SG, Rifkin A, Reardon GT (1982). Response of post-psychotic depression to adjunctive imipramine or amitriptyline. *Journal of Clinical Psychiatry, 43*(12): 485–486.

Siris S, Rifkin A, Reardon GT, Endicott J, Pereira DH, Hayes R, Casey E (1984). Course-related depressive syndrome in schizophrenia. *American Journal of Psychiatry,141*:1254–1257.

Siris SG, Rifkin A, Reardon GT, Doddi SR, Foster P, Straban A (1984). The dexamethasone suppression test in patients with post-psychotic depressions. *Biological Psychiatry,19*:1341–1356.

Siris SG, Rifkin A, Reardon GT (1985). A trial of adjunctive imipramine in postpsychiatric depression. *Pharmacology Bulletin, 21*:114–116.

Steidl J, Mandelbaum E (1987). Case studies and economics: Integrating a family-systems approach in adult medical settings. *Family Systems Medicine, 5*(2): 238–245.

Young AT (1987). Discharge planning and ethical dilemmas. *Discharge Planning Update, 7*(July/August):3–4.

1990s

Belville R, Indyk D, Shapiro V, Dewart T, Moss JZ, Gordon G, LaChapelle S (1992). The community as a strategic site for refining high perinatal risk assessments and interventions. *Social Work in Health Care, 16*(1):5–19.

Berrier J, Sperling R, Preisinger J, Mason J, Walther V (1991). HIV/AIDS education in a prenatal clinic: An assessment. *AIDS Education and Prevention, 3*(2):100–117.

Black RB, Weiss JA (1990). Genetic support groups and social workers as partners. *Health and Social Work, 15*(2):91–99.

Cincotta N, *et al.* (1990). *Radiotherapy Days*. Monograph. New York: Mount Sinai Medical Center.

Greenfield D, Walther V (1991). Psychological aspects of recurrent pregnancy loss. *Infertility and Reproductive Medicine Clinics of North America, 2*(1):235–247.

Mason J, Preisinger J, Sperling R, Walther V. (1991). Incorporating HIV education and counseling into routine prenatal care. *AIDS Education and Prevention, 3*(2): 118–123.

Rehr H (1991). An academic practice partnership in social work education. In C Irizarry, C James (Eds.). *Achieving Excellence in Health Social Work*. Adelaide, Australia: Flinders Press:85–96.

Showers N, Cuzzi L (1991). What field instructors of social work students need from hospital field work programs. *Social Work in Health Care, 16*(1):39–52.

Siegel ME, Greenspan E (1991). *Chemotherapy, Your Weapon Against Cancer*. Monograph. New York: Chemotherapy Foundation.

8

Community Development
and Lay Participation

Kenneth Peake, Barbara Brenner, and Gary Rosenberg

INTRODUCTION

The increasing complexity and changing relationships between health care providers and consumers are contributing to new and expanded roles for health care professionals, auxiliary health personnel, and consumers of health services. Lay participation in ongoing deliberations about health care delivery and quality within and outside the medical institution has begun to evolve into a partnership with providers. In that partnership, a community board gives voice to the individual needs of the consumer and the community at large.

A medical institution must be a product of its times. Its professionals, programs, and services must reflect the concerns, and respond to the demands of society, particularly to the people who live in the region in which they serve. Reeling under multiple pressures, especially economic ones, medical institutions must continually review their services and their delivery of care. To ensure that they maintain a positive place in their communities, medical institutions' missions must relate to their communities and residents through a partnership that leads to understanding individual and community needs and the development of sound solutions to problems.

"A university medical center must permanently concern itself with two groups of people, not just one. It must concern itself with its traditional constituency: the individuals who seek its help, as individuals, each year. And it must concern itself with its community, which may or may not be immediately adjacent to it, and which contains at any one time far more people who are well than who are not. The center must concern itself with these two groups. What it does for them, the ways it does it, and even the ultimate purposes of what it does are quite different" (McDermott, 1969).

But what is "a community?" Communities differ—in population, power structure, social structure, government structure, mental and emotional patterns, ethnic makeup, mores, religious and nutritional traditions, education, institutions, and organization. They differ in their prejudices and their prides, in their admixtures of poverty and wealth, in what they lack and in their abundances.

To work with a community demands multiple skills on the part of the caregivers. In assuming a relationship with the community, a medical center calls upon its various departments and its many providers who interact with consumers in a variety of ways. But these providers are governed by rules and regulations for the performance of services, and the rules sometimes impede their ability to facilitate the patient encounter. It is not uncommon for a department to act autonomously in a program designed for a community group, which can lead to fragmentation because the program has not been integrated with other services in the institution.

Consumers find it more and more difficult to make sense of labyrinthine health care systems and specialized, yet fragmented health care services. Getting access to and negotiating the labyrinth can be overwhelming, stressful, and full of contradiction. Access may be the single, most complex dynamic affecting prospective users and providers. Access not only refers to the ability to get care (i.e., crossing the threshold when needed; overcoming institutional barriers), but also refers to continuity in care and prevention of disease.

Large urban medical centers began as charitable care centers responsive to the particular conditions in the local communities from which they sprang. Community and psychosocial aspects of care were central to the missions of those institutions. Today, communities view large urban medical centers with suspicion—as wealthy, highly-specialized, monolithic entities that do not necessarily have the interests of the community at heart.

Most urban medical centers no longer serve only the culturally and ethnically homogenous populations from a well-defined geographical area. Because they are tertiary care institutions, usually with a range of specialized services, their patients come from far and wide. Primary care and satellite programs, however, are open to and used essentially by local community residents. With mandates to assure access to care for those in need, professional staff, particularly social workers, have attempted to be responsive to the local community. In some institutions this has been managed most effectively by including community representatives and agencies as partners in planning for and coordinating efforts to improve health care in the host communities. Often, however, barriers to partnerships exist and must be overcome before those partnerships can be effective.

BARRIERS TO PARTNERSHIP

DEFINITION OF PARTNERSHIP

Perhaps the first barrier to identify and overcome is that of definition. Dismissing for the moment the legal requirements of partnerships, of which there are some within the institution, in 1990s' parlance a partnership is a strategic alliance involving a close relationship between parties that have specified, joint rights and responsibilities. A partnership may by its very nature involve a degree of tension, as both parties in the partnership seek to ensure their rights, often, in their anxiety about rights and needs, ignoring responsibilities. This tension and consequent focus on rights is a barrier to achieving those rights, unless the definition also includes agreement regarding the central, shared purpose and focus of the partnership, thereby making clear each partner's responsibilities. With this in mind, it is clear that the urban medical center faces a number of dilemmas in any effort to define and/or create partnerships with its various communities, particularly within the immediately surrounding, external community and its community-based organizations.

TERRITORIALISM AND CONTROL

These two barriers are the byproducts of a competitive society, exacerbated by the fact that resources are strained to the limit. We compete for recognition for ourselves and our departments, often "rewriting history" in the quest for such recognition. We compete for funds to protect or sustain our own programs or pet projects, sometimes to the unfortunate demise of another critical program or project. We protect our own personal sources of income and advancement to the detriment of others. We foster fragmented activities or thwart progress toward effective planning to control the balance of power within a system. The politics of the system takes on a life of its own, and he who plays the politics cleverly broadsides the political neophytes. Somewhere, while we are all protecting our own turf, whether it be internal or external to the institution, the reason for our existence—the patient and community—is lost.

LACK OF COMMUNICATION

This particular barrier occurs in many forms, ranging from lack of effective communication and agreement within the institution regarding mission, purpose, and goals and objectives to an inability to listen to and hear what the internal and external communities are trying to communicate, and variations in between. While numerous organizational groups and a plethora of print media may exist, they may not be effective if the information from the former is not being acted on and the message within the latter is not absorbed. The hospital must have a pipeline to the community. Moreover, while the magnitude of groups, coalitions, boards, and committees may be great and representation significant, effective communication may not exist if other barriers, such as turfism and lack of clarity, exist.

Barriers to effective partnerships will exist unless there is vigorous leadership at critical levels within and outside the institution, inculcating a value system and culture that supports effective internal and external partnerships. Barriers will also exist unless there is systematic, integrated strategic planning, in which every action, every new program, every new investment fits the future that the hospital and its community have defined. In addition, barriers will exist if the medical center perpetuates or does not counteract its perception in the community as an elitist monolith that has forgotten its origins. For the urban medical center to rediscover its origins in, philosophy of, and commitment to community service, it must reexamine its existing programs, services, departments, and internal and external partnerships. It most likely will find that it already has built a foundation on which it can enhance existing community partnerships and build innovative new programs for the future.

THE RELEVANT LITERATURE

How has the social work professional responded to an increasingly specialized and complex health care system? Do hospital social workers define themselves in specialized ways or are they able to maintain a holistic view of their role in health care? Social work writings about community and lay participation demonstrate social workers' involvement and response to the need for partnership in two broad areas: 1) facilitation of access and responsiveness to the needs of the local community through development of partnerships with community agencies and groups; and 2) consumer empowerment through their involvement with providers and institutions in shared deliberations about the delivery and the quality of health services.

EXPANDING ROLES

The social worker has long held the role of "social broker" (Lamb, 1980; Wilson, 1981), which is assisting clients and consumers in negotiating complex, fragmented social service and health systems. The social broker function can greatly offset the tendency of social and health systems to disorient the consumer and fragment his care. Today the concept of the social broker can be expanded to include assisting consumers to obtain and interpret information that helps them make informed decisions about their health.

To remain effective, hospital social workers have had to define patient needs within the context of the hospital system and its many and varied professional and specialist groups. Their role has expanded and grown to incorporate the role of health educator and facilitator for the health system and its services. They demonstrate that social workers viewed the patient first as client and now as consumer "in sickness and in health." Simultaneously, they see other health professionals and the health care system as their clients, working in collaboration to further understanding of consumers' needs. Social workers interpret, "repackage," and publish information in a manner designed to help consumers understand complex health issues and enhance access to health care through consumer education. They bring a holistic approach to medical care, enhancing the quality and comprehensiveness of that care.

INNOVATIVE PARTNERSHIPS

Social workers long have defined community need as critical to the interests of the institution. They have initiated many innovative responses to the community, including service partnerships with community organizations. For example, an auxiliary board became a link between the board of trustees and the community, the first lay persons' liaison to the formal components of the medical institution—the "voice" of the consumer.

An early article written by a social worker about community and lay participation was published in 1957. Significantly, it presented the development of a program to enhance the auxiliary board's understanding of social casework to achieve its support for social work services. During this period social workers were concerned with establishing legitimacy within the institution. Some members of the auxiliary board also were members of the board of trustees, so enhancing an influential lay committee's understanding of psychosocial aspects of patient care and the impact of such factors on wellness and recovery became central to a long-term strategy.

The program consisted of case presentations carefully selected to communicate, in lay language, the spectrum of social work functions, which were described and defined in terms of patient needs. Careful orientation to, and understanding of casework methods were objectives of the presentations. Although the nature of the presentations evolved to include epidemiological studies, needs assessments, continuous quality assurance, and other broad-based, data-driven methods, the program of lay education has remained throughout the decades a vehicle for maintaining the visibility of social work and for innovative program development for the institution.

COMMUNITY BOARD

A community board was established in the 1960s during a period when the government recognized the need for community participation in reviewing its health care needs. Federal support of the Model Cities programs was responsible for early community involvement in hospital affairs. During the 1970s social workers described their collaborative enterprises with their health care professional colleagues. One revisited the work with the auxiliary board and described a presentation to educate the committee on the need for continuity of health care in the immediate posthospitalization period. Although the article emphasized patients' aftercare needs, it also highlighted the ongoing effort to maintain visibility, legitimacy, and support for social work services.

These articles, in which social workers collaborated with other health professionals, describe interagency collaborative planning between the medical center and community agencies. One described an agency network formed to improve access to health care for Medicaid-eligible families. Another outlined the development of a collaborative team comprised of medical center and community agency personnel, established to address health-related problems in community schools. These articles recognized that existing community organizations and schools, working in partnership with medical centers, can offset the fragmentation and disorganization that plague poor, inner-city communities, and that interagency coordination is an effective way to enhance access to health care for underserved groups.

Through the years, as a result of continued communication on the community board among consumer and provider members and of experience within the medical center, this small band of individuals has become better educated about medical center issues and health care and financial issues, and they have thus become able spokesmen and spokeswomen *about* the medical center. They also have taught each other—consumer-to-provider and provider-to-consumer—a significant amount about their individual issues and concerns. Each has used data from the other to solve problems internally and externally.

The medical center perceives a tremendous value added by the community board, in its activities, and in its actions and impact since inception. The internal community board has been an essential mechanism for ensuring that the medical center stays grounded in its social commitment to the community—an internal watchdog for signals that the medical center is straying from its mission; its members, for example, are aware of and vocal about consumer perceptions of the medical center, aware of and vocal about signs and symptoms of racial prejudice within the medical center, and vocal about ensuring a one-class system of care within the institution.

CONSUMER MODEL OF CARE

The 1980s produced a broader, less incremental institutional response to the relationship between the hospital and the community. In part this was a response to the rapid expansion and redevelopment of the hospital, increasing state mandates, and local demands for community involvement in planning and coordinating health care systems. In 1985 a social worker was appointed director of the department of community relations. The 1980s also saw increased interest in the consumer. Social workers embraced a consumer model of care, predicated on professional accountability to the client and concern for issues of client compliance and drop-out from services.

During this time, social workers addressed community and lay issues in their reflections on the widening arena of hospital social work in relation to communities and individual consumers. They presented frameworks for understanding the changing relationship between hospitals and users. In particular, they addressed social work issues in health care and performed a comprehensive examination of the consumer as user of health services and of consumerism on behalf of health care. The relationship between the consumer and provider in health care is described as a complex dynamic that affects client motivation, utilization of health care, and compliance with therapeutic regimes. During the late 1970s considerable interest was expressed in the issue of the "congruence" or fit between patient and professional understanding of treatment, including the role expectations that each had of the other (Orlinsky & Howard, 1986; Greenberg & Pinsof, 1986).

The concept of congruence was used to develop models for understanding and measuring patient satisfaction. Social workers sought to help patients address problems and concerns and enhance their future ability to cope. They wished to empower clients by developing their independent problem-solving skills. They helped develop patient self-help groups to manage social-medical problems and improve consumer participation through patient advocacy and consumer groups. Another major interest was in community relations and development. A third was in patient representation and patient rights' advocacy as institutional responsibilities. The concept of a community health ombudsman as the consumer's complaint bureau was initiated.

PROVIDER COLLABORATION WITH AGENCIES

The increasing awareness of the importance of community and lay participation in the medical center emerged during the 1970s. Social workers not only provided the conceptual framework for these emerging forms of community and lay participation, but helped consumers write their roles and participate in partnership programs with community agencies.

Provider collaboration with community agencies continued during the 1980s. The collaboration between a social worker and physicians described a joint effort between the medical institution and a nonprofit community agency that operated health services. The intent was to improve primary care enrollment and safeguard access to care for unserved community members with health problems. Despite initial success, however, difficulties at the governmental level in securing a change in the reimbursement system prevented successful implementation. The partnership effort failed because it was unable to overcome these external constraints.

A partnership that has continued is a multiprofessional collaboration in a successful program to reduce perinatal risk for a high-risk community population. A community agency was the primary source of service and drew on its expertise in working with multiproblem families in the immediate community. The agency demonstrated how essential its role was to the success of the partnership.

THE PRESENT

In the early 1990s social workers wrote about the linkages and partnerships they developed with diverse community groups and organizations, both in the immediate community and in the larger community served by the medical center. These linkages continue and represent a shift for social workers in health care as they move, with their professional colleagues, from providing essentially in-hospital services to providing a full range of social-health services on behalf of community residents. Returning to a community-organization model based on the settlement house movement, social workers will function in the community—providing health education, promotion and protection; supporting health maintenance; and drawing on high social-risk screening techniques to identify vulnerable populations. These efforts will occur in partnership with community residents, social agencies, and members of the medical center.

Although social workers will continue to serve the severely ill, those in crisis and those with acute care needs, they also will work with their partners to influence funding sources and assure data-gathering, preventive services, and identification of vulnerable populations.

In this era of fiscal crisis, cutbacks in government funding for community social-health projects, and the limited commitment of managed care companies to public health and care of noninsured persons, medical centers have found that limited resources impede their efforts in their communities. The current patterns of the service industry via its managed care policies, is to validate prevention as a benefit but to deny the provision for it. While public health agencies were set up to deal with prevention and health promotion, managed care companies have "skimmed" the Medicare and Medicaid patients, thus leaving public health facilities with limited or even no resources so that services are fast diminishing. In addition, the impact of illegal aliens and an increase in the marginal (noninsured) population has further eroded the public health mission.

The public will need to voice its concern with the emerging deficiencies in health care delivery. Policy deliberations by regional community partners focusing on their community social-health needs will be the major avenue to safeguard and to develop essential services. The medical center will be a participant, overcoming its barriers and citing the real and potential resources needed to effectively meet documented needs. In addition to delivery of care and preventive services, the medical center has a developing and a current knowledge and information base with which it needs to inform its local community, the public health and social agencies for regional community service planning.

The emphasis of collaboration is on being *with* the community rather than *for* them. By recognizing that social health problems are complex, by focusing on the locality—the neighborhood—it is possible to respond to needs in a comprehensive manner (Harkavy & Pucket, 1994; p. 309). The "locale" approach suggests a system of community service centers that is available to all residents and is comprehensive, accessible, and accountable. While factors of autonomy enter into downsizing, programs to create the one-stop center, an integrated network of services, collaborative and coordinated, could meld a biopsychosocial environmental approach to care, health promotion, and prevention.

If social workers are to be the link between medical centers and the community, they will need to influence the attitudes and behaviors of institutional leaders "to develop the capacity within their institution to reach out to learn about the strengths, needs, and dreams of their communities; help these institutions develop the capacity to respond to the needs of their communities by distilling knowledge, linking with others, engaging in an efficient collaborative planning program; initiate comprehensive programs; increase the accountability of institutions; and increase citizen control" (Chavis 1993; pp. 172–173).

In a changing health care environment, social work must reexamine its role in relation to the community. It must broaden its scope from an individual client perspective to community social-health orientation. Such expansion requires fostering meaningful collaboration with community residents and social-health agencies to:

- understand the community's social-health status;
- identify health and social needs, the gaps in service, and the programs essential to meet them;
- optimize availability of and accessibility to services;
- draw on social-epidemiological methods to screen for vulnerable populations and provide primary prevention;
- contribute to social-health planning efforts;
- further the understanding of public policy as it affects funding and service delivery;
- create a network of social-health services to allow for comprehensive care, including information and referral services for the local populace.

CONCLUSION

From the early 1950s, social workers demonstrated a recognition of the need to educate and inform a wide audience of consumers. Social workers have been leaders and participants in a wide array of efforts to broaden community and lay participation in health care. They have been involved extensively in developing planned partnerships with the community and have led efforts to develop institutional structures to support those partnerships. They led efforts to enhance consumerism to contribute to assessment and advocacy of quality health services. They used an array of vehicles to reach consumers, including journals, books, popular magazines and newsletters. They consistently raised awareness of issues of major significance to patients that had previously been neglected. They sought to empower consumers of health care through self-help and advocacy groups. Social workers have thus maintained and broadened the legitimacy and visibility of the profession while continuing their long-standing commitment to empower consumers and communities.

Like many academic health centers in urban settings, the medical center has traditional roles steeped in clinical, research, and education imperatives. However, like all voluntary, not-for-profit hospitals, it also has roots in community service, a strong commitment to social-health values, and a long history of community involvement; its staff and departments are directly or indirectly involved in an extensive number of community health programs, projects, committees, and groups. It has the people, the programs, and tools in place to effectively serve its communities. But existing capabilities must be enhanced and expanded to bring about more effective partnerships with and collaborative activities within the community. These capabilities need to be effectively connected within the medical center, with a particular group or department serving as the primary link between the community and the medical center as well as within the medical center, particularly for the review and consideration of new or revised programs and services, and how they will affect the community.

An internal community board, with its consumer and provider membership, could offer greater linkage with and communication between the medical center and the community. As a primary linkage within the medical center, the community board would be seen by provider and administrative staff members as an opportunity to forge a new community partnership and increase their own participation in shaping the mission of the hospital vis-a-vis the community. Increased communication between and linkage with the departments of community relations and the department of community medicine, through representatives on the community board, would be essential. An internal community board could also contribute to evaluation of the effectiveness of medical center community programs and could have more contact with other boards, community groups, and coalitions within the community in order to accomplish such an evaluation answering such questions as: Are programs effective? Are resources allocated appropriately? Do opportunities exist for redistribution of resources or realignment of focus?

And, finally, it is essential that community board activities and actions be routinely communicated to the board of trustees through formal, written minutes and that the community board be perceived in a proactive, rather than reactive role vis-a-vis the medical center and the community.

Commitment to community partnerships must start with the leadership of the institution and of the community. The renewed values of community commitment must be inculcated in every internal relationship/partnership. The urban medical center must rethink jobs, operating systems, and facilities in terms of it community commitment. It must move from competitive, fragmented planning to formal, integrated planning that is also flexible enough to quickly permit change when change is indicated. It must manage its resources—human, financial, technical, and organizational—proactively and ethically, and it must enlist the community for whom these resources exist to understand the responsibility we all have to use our resources prudently and wisely, targeting the needs of those we serve.

MOUNT SINAI REFERENCES

COMMUNITY DEVELOPMENT AND LAY PARTICIPATION

1960s

Rehr H, Goodrich C (1969). Problems of innovation in a hospital setting. In WC Richan (Ed.). *Human Services and Social Work Responsibility*. Silver Spring, MD: National Association of Social Workers, Inc.:303–309.
White E (1961). The role of the community in rehabilitation. *Social Casework*, July.

1970s

Berkman B (1977). Innovations for delivery of social services in health care. In F Sobey (Ed.). *Changing Roles in Social Work Practice*. Philadelphia, PA: Temple University Press.
Bosch S, Merino R, Daniels M, Fischer E, Rosenthal M (1979). A proposed network to improve access to high-quality health care for medicaid-eligible families. *Journal of Community Health*, 4(4):302–311.
Daniels M, Bosch S (1978). School health planning: A case for interagency collaboration. *Social Work in Health Care*, 3(4):457–467.
Paneth J (1972). Deflation in an inflationary period: Some current social health need provisions. *American Journal of Public Health*, January:60–63.
Rehr H (1972). Mount Sinai's social services in East Harlem. In *Proceedings: A Health Care Plan for East Harlem Now—Annals of the New York Academy of Sciences*, 196(2):80–81.
Rosengarten L, Paneth J (1977). How we communicate: A case presentation to a hospital auxillary board. *Social Work in Health Care*, 2(3):311–317.

1980s

Blumenfield S, Morrison B, Stroh J, Fizdale R (1981). The elderly and the social health care continuum. *Mount Sinai Journal of Medicine*, 48(6):569–572.

Daniels M (1980). Social work practice and community health: A planning implementation model. *Social Work in Health Care, 6*(2):39–51.

Dietch HH (1981). Community health ombudsman. In MD Mailick, H Rehr (Eds.). *In the Patient's Interest: Access to Hospital Care.* New York: Prodist:51–66.

Gruber T (1980). Ensuring that the system serves the patient. In DR Heacock (Ed.). *A Psychodynamic Approach to Adolescent Psychiatry: The Mount Sinai Experience.* New York: Marcel Dekker:305–309.

Lurie A, Rosenberg G (1984) (Eds.). *Social Work Administration in Health Care.* New York: Haworth Press.

Ravich R (1981). The advocacy role and education for patient representation. *Responding to the Health Care Consumer.* Monograph. U.S. Office of Consumer Affairs:44–51.

Ravich R (1986). Patient advocacy. In J Marks (Ed.). *Advocacy in Health Care.* Clifton, NJ: Humana Press:51–60.

Rehr H (1983). The consumer and consumerism. In R Miller, H Rehr (Eds.). *Social Work Issues in Health Care.* Englewood Cliffs, NJ: Prentice Hall, 2:20–73.

1990s

Belville R, Indyk D, Shapiro V, Dewart T, Moss JZ, Gordon G, LaChapelle S (1991). The community as a strategic site for refining high perinatal risk assessments and interventions. *Social Work in Health Care, 16*(1):5–19.

Young AT (1991). Social work practice with adolescent health and teenage pregnancy. In S Bardfield, RB Black (Eds.). *Social Work Practice with Maternal and Child Health: Populations at Risk, a Casebook.* New York: Columbia University School of Social Work:17–25.

9

Social Work Journalism: A Means to Consumer Health Education

Myrna I. Lewis and Mary Ellen Siegel

THE CONCEPT OF SOCIAL WORK JOURNALISM

Social workers writing for the public on health or other social issues bring a unique expertise and point of view to consumer health education. The authors have applied the term "social work journalism" to convey that uniqueness. Journalism as it traditionally is defined is the direct presentation of facts or "news" of current interest and wide, popular appeal, most often in newspapers, magazines, radio, and television. Health (or medical) journalism focuses more narrowly on the health and medical aspects of news; for example, medical or biological research findings, clinical innovations in the diagnosis and treatment of disease and disability, and updates on threats to the health of individuals and populations.

Social work journalism in the field of health care brings the knowledge, values, and traditions of the social work profession to the field of health journalism, most specifically, a biopsychosocial focus that is concerned with the whole person and with improving the ability to function optimally in one's environment. Health reporting and consumer education are combined to that end. Ideally, the social work health journalist combines writing skills with a knowledge of personality, interpersonal relations, physical and mental disease and disability, community resource availability, and prevention and health maintenance procedures in an effort to address sickness and health in a holistic, person-centered manner.

Social workers occupy two unique roles in relation to social work journalism. The first role carries a responsibility to consumers for their

117

health care maintenance and for quality health care. The goal is to give health care consumers the opportunity for autonomy and appropriate self-care, informed decision making, and collaboration with their health care providers.

The second role is a responsibility toward social work's professional health care colleagues. In this capacity, social workers address their health care partners about the need to support patients and family members through wellness and health education directives that enhance prevention, motivation, and compliance with patient care.

With both the consumer and the provider the focus is on understanding disease entities, information resources, and available support systems as well as reaching a partnership between provider and consumer.

THE EVOLUTION OF CONSUMER
HEALTH EDUCATION

Attention to the whole person, once dismissed as a romantic notion, is now emerging, transformed and renamed, as a central concept in health care, led by fields of practice such as geriatrics ("comprehensive geriatric assessment" and "case management"), and in the form of a team approach and humanistic medicine in a number of health care specialties.

This broader view of health care has been fueled by the consumer health or "self-help" movement that gained momentum in the 1980s and 1990s. Self-help activities sprang up around major medical diagnostic categories, where formerly the only recourse for patients had been to wait, worry, and wonder if their doctors could cure them. Cancer, heart disease, Parkinsonism, kidney dialysis, arthritis, AIDS, and sexual impotence—to name a few—are arenas in which patients became more informed and active participants in their own treatment.

Health care providers, initially often dubious about greater patient involvement, began to recognize that patient education could lead to better diagnoses, more appropriate treatment plans, better patient compliance with treatment, better outcomes, and greater overall patient satisfaction. By means of self-help and health education measures that included books and other print media, radio, television, videos, support groups, public seminars, and a growing dialogue between patients and their providers, self-help and consumer health education have helped the public acquire a sense of empowerment about their health, rather than assume the more passive position of patient or victim of disease.

An increased awareness of the importance of wellness rather than a focus on disease recovery brought further urgency to the concept of self-help. Older people and their health care providers began to realize that many of the diseases of later life are preventable or at least retardable. The middle-aged learned that remedies for the stresses of midlife were effective if one took the time to learn and apply them, and that physical and mental fitness have both immediate and long-term payoffs.

Baby-boomers, especially female baby-boomers who already were a huge, activist group of consumers, began to take health care into their own hands. One of the first targets was the childbirth experience: women focused on reexamining and transforming medical approaches to accommodate women's preferences and point of view. Later, an appraisal of menopause began, which rapidly changed public image, medical care, research, and self-help around this universal life event for females. Many predict that the same pattern of health care scrutiny and change, led by women health activists, will emerge in geriatrics and the health of the elderly as boomers find themselves growing older.

Managed health care companies are new players in the redefinition of health care—with an unforseen but interesting impact on the concept of self-help. Social work psychotherapists working on managed care health panels report that the brief therapy now almost universally required by managed care insurers in the interest of cost-savings can be bolstered with the use of reading lists, pamphlets and other educational tools to help clients learn self-treatment after their short interlude in formal therapy. Further, insurers are recommending that patients be regularly referred to low-cost or no-cost self-help, consumer education, and support groups in the community for any longer-term "group-work" necessary to address medical and/or psychological problems.

All of this has led to seemingly insatiable hunger on the part of the public for consumer health information and to a demand for writers who can translate health knowledge into a form understandable to the average lay person. Some of the focus areas include the latest medical research findings, physical and mental health treatments, knowledge of prevention of illness, treatment alternatives and self-treatments, and preservation and enhancement of personal wellness. The impact of social and psychological factors are critical areas of interest; people want to know how they can gain a greater sense of control and satisfaction over their own lives and assist those about whom they care. The management of relationships and the problems of communicating with others are central not only to personal emotional health but to physical health as well, with a growing body of medical research supporting this view.

HISTORY OF THE USE OF "BIBLIOTHERAPY"
IN CONSUMER HEALTH EDUCATION

Bibliotherapy is defined as "healing by means of the printed word." The term is usually used to refer solely to books. The authors have broadened the definition to include any form of journalism that focuses on providing health information to the public, including magazine and newspaper articles, health pamphlets, informational handouts, broadcast scripts, and health training materials that can be used by both health professionals and the general public (an example of the latter is the multipurpose information available on Alzheimer's disease). The "healing" aspects of bibliotherapy also have been broadened to encompass the *prevention of illness*.

Bibliotherapy has been used in the clinical practice of psychotherapy since at least the early part of the century—most prominently by the Drs. Karl and William Menninger who recommended bibliotherapy to their patients as a therapeutic tool (Bernstein, 1983). The practice of using "guided reading" (another term for bibliotherapy) has increased, especially in recent years (Katz & Watt, 1992; McKee, 1989; Quackenbush, 1991; Smith & Burkhalter, 1987; Starker, 1986, 1988). Pardeck focused on encouraging the practice of bibliotherapy in clinical social work (Pardeck & Pardeck, 1987; Pardeck, 1991). Siegel wrote of her own observations as a social worker about the value of bibliotherapy (Siegel, 1993). The use of bibliotherapy in specific interventions such as treatment of panic (Gould, 1993), cancer (Pardeck, 1992), and sexual and marital problems (Althof & Kingberg, 1992) has been described. A literature has grown up around the creation of consumer resource reading centers for diseases such as cancer (Eddleman & Warren, 1994; Watson, Medale, & Turman, 1994) and for general hospital use (Eisenstein and Faust, 1986). Studies of the efficacy of bibliotherapy also are making their way into the literature (Scoggin, Jamison, & Davis, 1990; Scoggin, Jamison & Gochneaur, 1989). Finally, studies of mental health topics in popular periodicals are revealing the popularity of the subject (Wahl, 1992).

In general, it is safe to say that although a modest portion of the public's reading on health-related subjects is guided by health professionals, the vast majority of such reading is self-guided—a form of self-therapy stimulated and initiated by browsing through bookstores, grocery store check-out shelves, magazine and paperback book racks, newspapers, the Internet, subscription magazines and newsletters, book reviews, and by following the reading recommendations of family, friends, and acquaintances. A range of health writing is called for, from the simplest, aimed at those with the lowest reading levels, along a continuum to a well-informed and highly literate audience.

THE UNIQUE ROLE OF SOCIAL WORK
IN HEALTH JOURNALISM

An article addressed to psychologists warns: "If we, who are trained and experienced in human behavior, fail to write the self-help books that people need, then by default they will be written by people with *less* training and experience. Our best assurance as psychologists that psychological self-help books are well written is to write them ourselves!" (Halliday, 1991; p. 680). The same could be said for social work in consumer education. If members of the social work profession fail to write for the public—not only books but a whole array of health education literature—a unique voice will be lost in consumer health care education. Williams and Hopps (1987) argue that writing and publishing are associated with professional maturity and the efficacy of a profession and that, by supporting social work values and human liberation, publishing serves a number of vital ends for the profession, the consumer, and the public in general. Social work traditionally has been the profession teaching the down-to-earth stance of "starting where the client is." This involves active interest in and understanding of varieties of people and a willingness to collaborate with them, starting *where they are.* A working partnership with the patient/client flows naturally from this stance, a partnership that translates into a straightforward communication style which ideally exhibits a special sensitivity and respect for the integrity, interests, and concerns of consumers.

Another social work precept especially useful to health journalism is the biopsychosocial approach discussed earlier. This daunting term simply extends the idea of holistic health care one step beyond its usual meaning involving the interconnections among mind, body, and emotions to include consideration of the individual's place in the family, community, society, and culture—the social part of the picture that surely and profoundly affects physical and emotional health.

In this connection, social work has another strength with a potentially powerful impact on consumer health education—namely its close identification with those most often left stranded on the fringes of the health care system—the AFDC mother and her children, the marginally employed, the poor elderly, the mentally ill, the homeless, the addicted, the many who cannot afford health insurance, and others. Much health literature for the public is directed toward the middle rather than the lower-income strata of United States society. Social workers can and should work to bring a balance to that literature, making certain that those most often excluded are included in their journalism. Whenever possible, social workers should be involved in creating a self-help and health education literature for those limited by problems of literacy, foreign language barriers, poverty, poor health, and the ongoing struggles to survive in harsh environments.

THE JOURNALISTIC ASPECTS
OF SOCIAL WORK JOURNALISM

Success in social work journalism depends not only on the knowledge social work brings to consumer education but also on writing skills (and for freelancers, marketing skills), the expertise developed around a subject, and the interest that the public, or at least a part of the public has at a particular time for a particular subject. Like journalism in general, social work journalism must either tap into current public concerns or, through a combination of compelling writing style, fact-gathering, and analysis, make the case that a neglected subject deserves public attention. The following elements are central to developing a career that either includes or is totally devoted to social work journalism in consumer health education.

DEFINING AN AREA OF FOCUSED EXPERTISE

This involves finding an area of expertise that combines knowledge with personal interest and commitment. Examples are health writing for one gender or the other, for certain age groups, or for a specific health problem such as addiction.

ASSESSING AND DEVELOPING WRITING SKILLS

Strengths and weaknesses as a writer for the public must be assessed—along with correction of identified weaknesses. Dozens of books about learning to be a writer are available. Among the most useful are Strunk and White's *Elements of Style* (Latest Edition), Zinsser's *On Writing Well* (1980), and Elbow's *Writing with Power* (1981). Private or college-based writing courses also can be useful.

ASSEMBLING A NETWORK OF CONTACTS AND COLLEAGUES

The object of networking is to obtain mutual psychological support and referrals of work, to gather information on publishing, and to keep up-to-date on consumer health writing. A convenient way to begin to meet other writers is through organizations of writers, including the American Society of

Journalists and Authors, the Women's National Book Association, the International Women Writers' Guild, the American Medical Writers Association, the Author's Guild, and others. Membership in these groups usually is limited to those who already have published, although many groups offer open meetings which the interested public can attend.

LEARNING THE PUBLISHING FIELD

It is not enough to learn to write; one must also learn how to be published. *How to Get Happily Published* by Judith Appelbaum (1993), is one of the most current and comprehensive sources of information in this area. Book and/or magazine agents also need to be considered, especially for full-time journalists. Writers' conferences and symposiums, sponsored by writers' groups and universities can be very helpful. For example, the American Society of Journalists and Authors presented a symposium co-sponsored by the American Psychological Association, "Getting Published, Getting Known," designed to help mental health professionals educate the lay public through the public media. This symposium was held in New York City, and similar ones are conducted in other parts of the country. Participants learn how to develop articles and books, work with collaborators, and communicate with the media. For those unable to attend, audiotapes of sessions usually are made available.

Browsing through a large bookstore or library will also yield many good books that can serve as resources for those entering the field. Some mental health professionals might prefer to collaborate with an established writer who has contacts in the publishing field and who is more familiar with the way material should be presented.

USING RADIO AND TELEVISION AS A TEACHING FORUM

The broadcast media of radio and television are often the *only* way to reach the large health consumer audience that does little or no reading. Social work journalists not only write for the media, but also appear on radio and television as hosts, reporters, health care specialists, and advocates.

MOUNT SINAI SOCIAL WORK JOURNALISM

Social workers at Mount Sinai began to address consumer-related health education in the late 1970s with two articles—one addressed to professionals to help the consumers of medical care assume informed decision making, the second addressed to the lay public about how to cope with cancer. In the 1980s, social workers burst forth into social work journalism, as evidenced by works in monographs, chapters and books, newspapers and organization newsletters, and popular magazines.

The professional thrust in the 1980s was largely on the significance of geriatric issues such as elder abuse, the psychological aspects of terminal illness, understanding bereavement and grief following loss, and helping patients and families manage the treatment impact of chemotherapy or radiotherapy. Social workers also wrote of health educational programs with selected groups such as parents of chronically ill children, and also proffered detection and assessment tools to screen for social risk in medical situations as well as intervention strategies.

The other major thrust of writings in this period was addressed to the consumer and to professionals—demythologizing sexuality for aging persons. Articles and books focused on sexuality in mid- and later life. In addition, social workers wrote for the public on coping with the impact of physical disorders and illnesses with the emphasis on how to deal with different forms of cancer. A number of popular articles appeared in magazines and books on subjects such as hair loss, child care, drinking and gambling problems, and the problems of women as they age.

As the 1990s began, the pattern continued of addressing professionals in their own literature about health education as well as targeting the lay public through the popular media. Today social workers emphasize consumer health care needs and strategies for managing them. A new dimension has been introduced in this period as social workers advise the public on patient rights in the use of medical services.

CONCLUSION

Social work journalists in health care function as professionals who are both journalists/writers and social workers, bringing a body of social work knowledge and values to consumer health education. Their professional training in the dual areas of social work and health care enables them to act as demystifiers of health information for the health care consumer. The use of a wide range of media from print to broadcast journalism makes it feasible to reach the broadest possible public audience, much of the time at low cost or no cost to the consumer. Journalism also is an effective vehicle for social work advocacy around unpopular but important public health issues, such as the budget needs of vital social and health programs.

The goals of social work health journalism are synonymous with social work health care as a field, and consumer education as a specialty, namely to enable as many people as possible to make informed choices about and effective use of health care services, to promote self care and techniques for the prevention and moderation of disease and disability, and to help make possible a greater sense of personal mastery over the preservation of that most valuable of life's gifts—good health.

MOUNT SINAI REFERENCES

SOCIAL WORK JOURNALISM: A MEANS TO HEALTH EDUCATION

1970s

Butler RN, Lewis M (1976). *Love and Sex After Forty*. New York: Harper & Row. Revised edition, 1988.
Butler RN, Lewis M (1973). *Aging and Mental Health: Positive Psychosocial and Biomedical Approaches*. New York: C.V. Mosby. Revised editions, 1977, 1986, 1991 (with Sunderland T).
Dana B (1977). Consumer health education. *Proceedings of the Academy of Political Science*, 32(3):182–192.
Siegel ME (Kulkin) (1979, April). Cancer: There is hope. *National Council of Women of the United States, XXVI*.

1980s

Butler RN, Lewis M (1984). Sexuality and aging. *The Seicus Report*. Monograph. 12:12–13.
Butler RN, Lewis M (1987). Love in the land of old age. *The Washington Post: Weekly Journal of Health*, April.
Butler RN, Lewis M (Eds.) (1988). *Midlife Love Life: A Guide for Men and Women for Their Mid and Later Years*. New York: Harper & Row.
Cincotta N (1989). I'd rather be swimming. New York: Leukemia Society of America.
Greenberger M, Siegel ME (Eds.) (1980). *What Every Man Should Know About His Prostrate*. New York: Walker & Co:1–146.
Lewis M, Butler RN (1984). Why is women's lib ignoring old women. In M Minkler, CL Estes (Eds.). *Readings in the Political Economy of Aging*. New York: Baywood Publishers:199–208.
Lewis M (1985). Older women and health: An overview. In S Gould, R Freedman (Eds.). *Health Needs of Women as They Age*. New York: Haworth Press:1–16.
Lewis M, Osako M (1985). Conversation with a geisha. *Quarante: Magazine for the Woman Who's Arrived*, 33–39.
Lewis M, Butler RN (1985). The facts of later life. *Modern Maturity*, February/March:59–60.
Lewis M (1986). Advocacy Issues for Older Women. In JH Marks (Ed). *Advocacy in Health Care: The Power of a Silent Constituency*. Clifton, NJ: Humana Press:67–75.
Lewis M (1987). Sex bias dangerous to women's mental health. *Perspective on Aging*. National Council on Aging:9–12.
Lewis M (1988). Answers about aging: Sex after sixty. *National Institute on Aging Information Programs*, July:1–6.

Lewis M (1988). Global aspects of older women's lives. *International Forum/Joint (JDC) Israel Brookdale Institute of Gerontology and Adult Human Development.* Monograph. Jerusalem, Israel: Joint (JDC) Israel Institute of Gerontology and Adult Human Development:15.

Ravich R (1981). The advocacy role and education for patient representation. *Responding to the Health Care Consumer.* Monograph. U.S. Office of Consumer Affairs:44–51.

Rosengarten L (1986). Creating a health-promoting group for elderly couples on a home health care program. *Social Work in Health Care,* 11(4):83–92.

Siegel ME (Kulkin) (1980). Women demand adult treatment. *National Council of Women of the United States,* XXVII(5).

Siegel ME, Greenspan E (1980). The role of chemotherapy in the control and care of disseminated cancer. *Jewish Teachers Association Newsletter,* September.

Siegel ME (1982). Mature concerns. *Moving On, A Queens Community Newsletter,* March/October.

Siegel ME (1984). I can cope with cancer. *Cancer News,* Spring/Summer: 10–12.

Siegel ME, Koplin H (Eds.) (1984). *More Than a Friend: Dogs with a Purpose.* New York: Walker and Co.

Siegel ME (1985). *Reversing Hair Loss.* New York: S&S Trade.

Siegel ME (1986). Suffering: Psychological and social aspects in loss grief and care. In R Debillis, E Marcus, A Kutcher, C Torres, V Barrett, ME Siegel (Eds.). New York: Haworth Press.

Siegel ME (Ed.) (1986). *The Cancer Patient's Handbook.* New York: Walker and Co.

Siegel ME (1986). Hair loss is a loss. *Archives of the Foundation of Thanatology,* 12(4).

Siegel ME (1988). Children's reactions to death of grandparents and great grandparents: Case histories. In O Margolis, A Kutscher, E Marcus, HC Raether, VR Pine, I Seeland, D Cherico (Eds.). *Grief and the Loss of Adult Child.* New York: Praeger.

Siegel ME, Ferri E (1988). FingerTips. Appeared in *Ladies Home Journal, Modern Guide, Women's Day* and *Cosmopolitan.* New York: Crown Publishers.

Siegel ME (1988). *Psychiatric Aspects of Terminal Illness.* Philadelphia, PA: Charles Press.

Siegel ME (1989). Am I Pandora's keeper? *Archives of the Foundation of Thanatology,* 15(1).

Sweet AR, Siegel ME (Eds.) (1987). *The Nanny Connection.* New York: Atheneum Press.

Young AT (1980). *An Exploratory Study of the Educational Process of Parents of Chronically Ill Children: Diabetes and Asthma.* Dissertation. New York: Columbia University Teachers' College.

1990s

Berrier J, Sperling R, Preisinger J, Mason J, Walther V (1991). HIV/AIDS education in a prenatal clinic: an assessment. *AIDS Education and Prevention,* 3(2):100–117.

Butler RN, Lewis M (1990). Sexuality and aging. In WB Abrams, RW Berkow, AJ Fletcher (Eds.). *The Merck Manual of Geriatrics.* Rahway, NJ: Merck:632–642.

Cincotta N, *et al.* (1990). *Radiotherapy Days.* Monograph. New York: Mount Sinai Medical Center.

Mason J, Preisinger J, Sperling R, Walther V, Berrier J, Evans V (1991). Incorporating HIV education and counseling into routine prenatal care. *AIDS Education and Prevention*, 3(2):118–123.

Ravich R (1990). Patient's rights in breast surgery. In A Gross, D Soto (Eds.). *Women Talk About Their Surgery*. New York: Potter:300–307.

Ravich R (1991). Patient's rights in gynecological surgery. In A Gross, D Soto (Eds.). *Women Talk About Their Surgery*. New York: Potter:308–317.

Siegel ME (1991). Chemotherapy: A social work perspective. *Chemotherapy Foundation Newsletter* (Quarterly from 1980–1991).

Siegel ME, Greenspan E (1991). *Chemotherapy, Your Weapon Against Cancer*. Monograph. New York: Chemotherapy Foundation.

Siegel ME (1990). *Safe in the Sun*. New York: Walker and Co.

Siegel ME (1990). Rites of passage/rights of passage. In A Kutscher, S Bess, S Klagsbrun, ME Siegel, DJ Cherico, L Kutscher, D Peretz, FE Selder (Eds.). *For the Bereaved: The Road to Recovery*. Philadelphia, PA: Charles Press: 64–68.

Siegel ME (1990). What about me? Unrecognized and unsanctioned grief: The nature and counseling of unacknowledged loss. In V Pine, O Margolis, K Doka, A Kutscher, DJ Schaeffer, ME Siegel, DJ Cherico (Eds.). *Archives of the Foundation of Thanatology*. Springfield, IL: CC Thomas.

Siegel ME (1991). What every woman should know about ovarian cancer. *Coping: Living with Cancer*, 4:(Spring)29.

Simon EP (1990). The therapeutic companion program. *Archives of the Foundation of Thanatology*, 16(2).

10

Educating for Social-Health Care: Social Work Practitioners, Students, and Other Health Care Professionals

Helen Rehr, Gary Rosenberg, Virginia Walther,
Nancy Showers, and Alma Young

Two major trends in our society will have an impact on social work education in the future: the changing health care environment and its financing, and the changing demographics of society. Both cause education structures as they relate to the social work service delivery system to lag behind other structures.

THE CHANGING HEALTH CARE ENVIRONMENT

The United States is witnessing the most drastic industrial reorganization since the 19th century. The corporate takeover of American health care is a primary example of this trend upheaval. Giant health systems have been created, formed not by their own desires, but in the crucible of employer and insurer demands for lower costs and by a government unable to legislate health reform.

Businesses and governmental agencies that pay for health care have organized to force the insured population to use designated providers. By and large, patient freedom of choice has been exchanged for lower costs. The health care system will be influenced in the future by four characteristics that will affect the way systems operate:

1. The system will be vertically integrated. From preventive services, wellness programs, and health education through primary care,

secondary and acute care to long-term care, all services will be handled through one unified system.

2. Regional system coverage will replace local catchment areas as the dominant form of targeting patients, resulting in a wide geographic area of people being served.

3. Payment by capitation. The health care system will share the risks and potential rewards and will be paid a flat fee per covered life or per covered service/package.

4. Costs will be lowered below the present non-managed-care market prices.

To increase the scope of health care services while decreasing the costs, the new delivery system will require redeployment of major resources and people from inpatient acute care to ambulatory care, from specialist settings to primary care programs, and from tertiary care to early diagnosis and prevention.

Major changes in the health care delivery system have been affected by restructuring of the system itself. Because of fiscal concerns and the drive for higher levels of productivity, an increasing number of hospitals are restructuring, both by expanding to become health care systems, and by flattening the administrative structures of the system, thereby creating a horizontal system of management.

Changing the way work is done and eliminating unnecessary work are essential, but superfluous work must first be identified (Campy, 1995). To organize around core processes rather than functions, a concept borrowed from the business world, is the current central aim. In this organizational design, the health care environment is expected to be seamless, uncluttered by boundaries among departments where discontinuities can occur and where difficult and unnecessary work processes can appear (Bergman, 1995).

As a result of restructuring of the health care environment, health care professional groups have had to justify and redefine themselves to administrations and to each other. The professions maintain that practice expertise is specific and unique to each discipline and that organizations benefit from their centralization. Present-day system managers call for the removal of professional boundaries through cross-trained staff as one way to improve patient care and reduce costs (Ford & Randolph, 1992; Dimond, 1993). Which professional boundaries to keep has become an issue. To bridge such divergent perspectives, new structural models must be developed so that the values and concerns of the designs mesh with professional goals.

How does a profession maintain and control standards for quality professional practice, staff education, teaching, and research, and the development of innovative programs of care in the new health care systems? The challenge for social work is to enhance its educational base, drawing on changing organizational patterns of health care and on the integration of innovative practice, programs, and research. This tests practice and programs and advances behavioral and social science theories.

CHANGING DEMOGRAPHIC TRENDS

Among the most prominent demographic trends today are the changing nature of the family, the expansion of the population over 65, the growth in the numbers of children 11 years of age and under, and the rapid growth of out-of-wedlock pregnancies which have quadrupled since 1950 and represent 18.4% of all births. These and other demographic factors affect the focus and educational underpinnings of social work practice.

SOCIAL WORK SERVICE DELIVERY
AND ITS EDUCATION STRUCTURES

Social workers increasingly are realizing that practice wisdom and scientific technologies must be assessed together to identify ways in which social work services can be enhanced. Unfortunately, social work is a profession splintered into many component parts. For example, casework is separated from group work and community organization; the clinical area is separated from social policy; academics are separated from practitioners. Social work is not perceived as an entity but as an array of multiple and separate components that function independently. Moreover, disparate and controversial directions occur within each component. Each moves along its own pathway. Those in the clinical enterprise espouse different frames of reference/theory to support their practice, if theory is espoused at all. Some trained social workers go so far as to deny the profession while they seek a place among psychotherapists or in other behavioral modalities.

The splits drain our professional energy. Rather than find common ground or value from conflict, they contribute to reduced respect from and confusion among those outside the profession who observe our inexplicable differences. The social work educational structure tends to encourage compartmentalization.

"We in social work have borrowed our foundations from psychology, psychiatry, medicine, sociology and social psychology and have tried over the years to make something that is unique and our own. Such a quest, however worthy, may have been unrealistic. It is time to use that which is our own, the research conducted by social work professionals. Those responsible for social work education must apply those findings to social work's advantage for the sake of the profession's development of accountability, effectiveness and professional structure so that we may be ranked among other professional schools. Likewise, these research findings should be used to find solidity and a common core within the social work curriculum at all levels. The integration of theory, practice, and research has been difficult to achieve in social work education. Nevertheless, issues of accountability, ethical pressures and data on practice effectiveness provide the impetus for integration. It is time to stop questioning and criticizing and to apply the existing research to develop a rational framework among our many interests within the degree levels of social work" (Wodarske, Feit, & Green, 1995).

Although restructuring of health care organizations may eliminate the centralized structure of social work departments, the profession's influence on services and socialization of the institution *can prevail*. Social work's contribution to the institution's image and revenue base becomes critical. Creative partnerships between the field and its educational institutions are essential if social work is to maintain its role as an important health and mental health profession.

The contributions of empirical data to practice decisions are undeniably important, but on their own they provide an insufficient knowledge base for practice that is informed by multiple sources of information and a variety of thinking processes, including ideas, beliefs, intentions and attitudes derived from public culture (Berlin, 1990). The split has widened between psychotherapy based in psychiatry and the provision of social service. Social work in health is multidimensional; not only is it biopsychosocial but it is fully social-environmental as well. These dimensions are critical in shaping the future development of social work practice and they will affect the roles of research and education as the practice evolves (Epstein, 1995).

FUTURE DOMAINS IN SOCIAL WORK

Social work practice in health care will take place in the community as well as in the hospital. It will focus on the person and defined populations. It will be a mix of social service provision and short- and long-term counseling. It will take place in teams of multidisciplinary professionals and paraprofessionals. Although social work services might not be centralized in the traditional sense, they will be structured to influence social work practice and the institution as social workers form consortia or coalitions. Supervision as it is known today will not exist. Maintaining high standards of practice will require new modes of education and continuous learning. Social workers will need to be autonomous and self-directed.

PROGRAMS TO ENHANCE COMMUNITY HEALTH

Community health programs are based on the concept of developmental provision. Social work will help provide "those social utilities designed to meet the normal needs of people arising from their situations and roles in modern life" (Kahn, 1969). Social work along with other professions will help provide the social architecture for enhanced community living.

By the year 2000, the continuing shift to service occupations will play a major role in formulating disease patterns. The interaction of the increasing rate of change, shifts in technology, greater crowding (population density), information overload, and stress—all characteristics of the service and transformation society—will play a role in creating new disease patterns. Practice will be based on the concepts that:

- an integral relationship exists between people's health and their environment, to the extent that although confronting the actual infective and causative agents of disease is critical, it is secondary to changing the social and physical environmental conditions that permit disease onset;
- vulnerability to new waves of health risk is greater for the economically disadvantaged in every community in developed and developing countries, so that improvement in living conditions becomes, by definition, a social-health promotion strategy; and
- physical and social functioning of individuals in relation to their informal and formal networks is more significant than the disease pattern itself.

Through the use of social epidemiology and survey methods, health care social workers will be helpful in identifying and reducing health risks. As they contribute to health promotion, social workers will add to community strengths. In part, the move to this domain represents a return to our settlement house roots, which emphasized amelioration and reform from an empowerment perspective, social science as an integral part of practice, a comprehensive response to complex problems, and cross-functional program management. In this domain, social workers will:

- relate to the organization's mission, dealing with constraints while translating public policy into programs that focus on individual need;
- help institutional leaders develop the capacity to reach out to their communities and learn about their strengths, needs, and wants;
- help their institutions respond to the needs of their communities by identifying models, distilling research knowledge, linking the institutions with others that have similar dreams, brokering resources with other institutions, developing the social technologies to be tested and refined, and engaging in an efficient collaborative planning process;
- build the capacity of local institutions to initiate comprehensive programs;
- increase the accountability of institutions;
- increase citizen participation in and control over institutions; and
- define social work's role in the socialization of the institution.

INTERVENTION WITH VULNERABLE POPULATIONS

Numerous research studies have demonstrated that psychological, educational, and behavioral interventions in vulnerable populations are efficacious in a practical as well as in a collective sense. The vulnerable populations include minorities, the elderly, the chronically ill, and the chronically mentally ill.

MINORITIES

"By virtually every health status indicator—life expectancy, mortality, morbidity, and utilization of and access to health resources—minorities fare more poorly than the general population" (USDHHS, 1985). To use an example of specific geographic communities, the reported rate of survival beyond the age of 40 was lower for men in Harlem than for men in Bangladesh. The death rates per 100,000 population are higher in Harlem than in New York City as a whole for all causes combined as well as for AIDS, pneumonia and influenza, cerebrovascular disease, chronic obstructive pulmonary disease, chronic liver disease and cirrhosis, drug dependence, and accidental drug poisoning, homicide, and undetermined injuries.

The potential for improvement through increased prevention efforts appears vast.

THE ELDERLY

In 1900, the number of people over 65 constituted 4% of the population; by 2030 they will constitute 22% of the population. Older adults currently comprise 12% of the population of the United States and use one-third of physicians' time. They comprise 40% of hospital admissions, purchase 25% of medications sold, and account for 36% of personal health expenditures. The proportion who experience disability increases with age, to the point where almost "half of those 85 and older need assistance in activities of daily living." The estimated probability of using a nursing home increases as age of death increases—from 17% for those who die between 75 and 84 years of age to 60% for those who die between 85 and 94 years of age (US-DHHS, 1990). Services that support this vulnerable population and families wishing to support them are crucial.

THE CHRONICALLY ILL

In the United States, approximately "33 million people have functional limitations that interfere with their daily activities, and more than nine million have limitations that prevent them from working, attending school, or maintaining a household" (USDHHS, 1990). A growing population of chronically ill persons exists who, with advancing technology, will be able to receive care in ambulatory settings or in the home. Technologies for effective case management services and knowledge of the psychopharmacological and biochemical base of disease and its social consequences are, and will be, part of social workers' knowledge base.

THE CHRONICALLY MENTALLY ILL

Social workers will need to provide continuous psychosocial intervention for psychologically vulnerable populations. It will become increasingly essential for social workers to intervene directly in the family system, not only with the ill person but with caregivers. When family caregiving or social support is unavailable, as often is the case, social work must be equipped to integrate formal and informal systems of care. While social work will be conducted in traditional and nontraditional settings, the objectives of intervention always will be to reduce the years of mentally unhealthy life and enhance the years of mentally healthy life beyond medical notions of mental health as simply the lack of mental illness.

As we work with vulnerable populations, we must be vigilant against the medicalization of social services. Health promotion becomes more meaningful for understanding population, while medical care remains more significant for the individual sick. The most important determinants of health status are preventive services and quality of life standards.

EDUCATION OF SOCIAL WORK PRACTITIONERS

Professional social workers have a long history of self-education, of collaborating with other disciplines in education, and of encouraging and promoting education of volunteers, students in all the health professions, and the public. Early experience was translated into content; courses and structured educational programs subsequently were devised. The social work profession is responsible for:

- continuing the education of social work practitioners so they can offer services that are relevant to the social-health problems of the times;
- developing tomorrow's social work professionals through investment in collaborative partnerships with schools of social work and the provision of sound practice education in health care settings;
- transmitting social work values and knowledge to other health care professions in order to enhance their understanding of social-health concerns and service delivery; and
- educating others (e.g., volunteers) about the nature of social work services so that they can help make services available.

Social work also is responsible for health education efforts related to wellness, primary care, and health maintenance promotion for the general public and for projected populations-at-risk.

CONTINUING EDUCATION

Every professional social worker, regardless of field of practice or modality, requires continuing education to develop advanced social work practice, skill, and expertise. No field of service can remain constant or static; each must reorder its practices and priorities with societal and organizational changes. In their efforts to improve the quality of their service, agencies offer orientation for new employees and in-service training to inform practitioners about agency policies and programs and to enhance their knowledge base and practice skills. When linked to schools of social work, agencies often establish clinical relationships or research partnerships with academics. Continuing education is essential to all professions that serve the public because:

- new knowledge must be applied to practice concurrently; academic educational programs are the beginning, not the end of learning;
- maintaining currency in clinical content enhances professional status and state licensing and recertification should require upgrading knowledge;
- research and innovation in practice is stimulated by group learning;
- professional standards are promoted and revitalized;
- advanced learning improves economic potential; and
- vendor reimbursement levels are enhanced.

Continuing education is the responsibility of the individual social worker, the professional association, the professional department of social work, and the agency in which practice takes place. It is the bridge between professional performance appraisal in which areas for improvement are identified and program assessment in which recommendations for improvement have been applied.

PEER REVIEW AND CONTINUING EDUCATION

Social workers are effective in preventing the overuse (risk exceeds benefit), underuse (failure to use services), and misuse of health services. How do social work services add to the quality, effectiveness, and appropriate use of the health system? How does social work contribute to achieving a desired health outcome consistent with current professional knowledge? Social work has developed and implemented the following:

- high social-risk screening as part of standardized assessments;
- health social work protocols that standardize known treatment techniques that are proven effective; and
- information systems that capture and evaluate outcome data and provide feedback about effectiveness to providers and payers.

THE RELEVANT LITERATURE

Peer review (quality assurance) of social work practice was institutionalized and linked to continuing education as the need for more knowledge
and skill was uncovered through the peer review process or the direct request of practitioners. As early as 1959, when supervision was characterized
by its goal to enhance social work practice, the implied result of supervision was self-directed social workers. In the early 1960s, knowledge gained
from programs for poliomyelitis victims was translated into educational
content that informed social work practice for patients suffering from
chronic disorders. In particular, key treatment dimensions were: the significance of body image, the pivotal role of interprofessional collaboration,
and the need for community networking to enhance management of
chronic illness. An experiment involving both staff and administration in
planning resulted in an integrated, dynamic staff development program
for continuous improvement of practice. This was predicated on the belief
that practice and programs would require change over time in response to
a social-health evolution.

The conceptual base for self-directedness was drawn from the physician
model of peer review and organizational opportunities for enhanced learning. Peer review developed along professional standards set for achievement. To achieve the goal of producing self-directed workers, a joint staff-
administration project was initiated in the early 1970s with the design and
implementation of a major in-service training program that established
principles, guidelines, and programs for educational development within
the social work department. The self-directed worker was defined as one
who functions with an awareness of self and a commitment of accountability to the client system, the department, the medical institution, regulatory bodies, and the profession. The commitment calls for a continuous
reexamination of practice and continued enhancement of professional
knowledge.

As the quality assurance and continuing education program developed,
social workers agreed that participant evaluation of the program should
occur. In spite of recognized difficulties in formal assessment of behavior
and/or resultant program change, participant outcomes were measured
via satisfaction with the continuing education program and with perceived
professional gains as the staff assessed educational content and learning.

During the 1970s, professional standards review organizations, promulgated by the federal government to evaluate the quality of care for
Medicare and Medicaid recipients, expected professional accountability
for performance and program evaluation. The social work department

documented the delivery of social work services, including the who, what, and how of service delivery. Next, the department assessed outcomes of service. The development of problem classification, contractual agreements between clients and workers, and outcomes provided the means to assess the social work product and led to awareness of continuing education objectives. Chart documentation became a measurement tool to identify compliance with standards. Special programs were introduced to enhance learning, including a gerontology journal club (which addressed innovative content relevant to the elderly), a basic orientation program, and specialized tools for quality discharge planning as well as an in-service training program to develop research skills for practitioners. Group education was established as was individual, contracted supervision outside the formal administrative hierarchy using expert senior practitioners.

A review of publications reveals a substantial number that focus directly on supervision and continuing education. A majority of articles, no matter the topic, also address ongoing educational implications. A professionally accountable social work service that supports continuing education provides the basis for quality improvement in practice and in program. It also can effectively achieve its objective to educate social work students and other health care professionals.

SOCIAL WORK STUDENT EDUCATION

THE CHALLENGE

Academic social work education does not fully prepare professionals to work in the wide range of health care settings that exists today. It has done little to introduce health content or to emphasize health promotion and maintenance, primarily because faculty members have limited practice and health care experience.

To function effectively in health care practice settings, social workers must have current knowledge of the health care delivery system and must understand dynamic changes in the system and how to deal with them. To practice effectively in complex health care systems, social workers must understand the intricacies of the organizational structure, health care financing and its correlation with service delivery, and financing within the practice setting. Moreover, as social workers begin to practice in disease-specific arenas, knowledge of disease, disorders, and disability is required. As students, social workers must understand the direct and indirect im-

pact of illnesses on individuals, families, society, and themselves. The social and physical limitations that might be the consequences of illness and
of the individual's social environment are primary areas for patient and
family counseling to ensure optimum achievement of patient social-health
goals. Finally, the multiprofessional organization of social-health care demands skills in collaboration and team work.

To collaborate successfully requires professional self-realization, patient advocacy, and partnership with other health care professionals. Some
specialization in social work student education is therefore essential. Concentration on the social and physical implications of disease can be critical
to providing knowledgeable service to clients regardless of setting. Family-focused practice requires that social workers be able to perceive the impact of illness on family and to help secure family equilibrium. A working
knowledge of social-health diagnostic and therapeutic processes and relevant resources is key to service in any setting. Although new graduates are
not expected to be fully prepared to handle these complex situations, they
are expected to understand that sickness and medical care are phenomena
of daily living.

THE RELEVANT LITERATURE

The social work department has sustained an educational responsibility
for preparing tomorrow's professional social workers. Until the late 1960s
the role was maintained in traditional supervisor/student educational
modes. By the end of the 1960s, a fortuitous relationship between a staff
practitioner and a school of social work faculty member led to major change
in student education. An academic/practice partnership (a consortium of
one school and several affiliated health care settings) was created to prepare social work students to be effective new graduates. The primary curriculum objective was "to educate students to be professionally responsive
to the needs of people in changing patterns of care." The consortium expected that students master relevant skills and knowledge as well as develop collaborative skills, professional accountability, skills in program
administration, and a capacity to experience oneself in an interdependent
relationship with other professionals and community agencies.

The experience in promulgating the concept of a self-directed social
worker served as the cornerstone of the new educational partnership. The
use of group learning, multiple instructors as preceptors, and multiple
learning sites helped students develop a commitment to professional ac-

countability, prepare to be self-reliant, and value peers and experts as sources of ongoing learning. In addition to providing a structure for student education, the model contained rich potential for ongoing development of professional staff. As instructor preceptors developed skills in group education, they conceptualized practice, issues, system demands, and interprofessional collaboration, and assumed new teaching roles.

Two consequences of this innovative education partnership are noteworthy. First, graduates of the program were committed to the importance of continuing education and sought employment in agencies with strong continuing education programs. Secondly, many components of the educational design (e.g., multiinstructor and multisite learning opportunities) have been introduced in social work departments of other teaching hospitals and in schools of social work.

The social work department also undertook several other education projects. For example, professional associations sponsored two major literature reviews, one of which reviewed the literature for the clinical practice of social work in mental health and aging and a second which reviewed the knowledge base and program needs required for effective social work practice in health care. Both became useful research resources for related concentrations in academic programs.

A study of five affiliated hospital social work departments resulted in recommendations for student education of social workers and other health care professionals and led to several published articles about specific programs. These included special concentrations for students in counseling techniques—specifically a psychoeducational, family-focused model for mentally ill patients; an educational program that addressed how to establish the social work role in team collaboration; a curriculum to understand the constraints and benefits of a complex organization and how to work in the organization on a patient's behalf; a summer fellowship in gerontology for social work students to enhance knowledge and address the skills needed to work with older persons; training in practice-research, also introduced as a special concentration; and shared educational objectives for social work and medical students.

An early article described an instrument to assess social work student education in the hospital setting. The evaluation tools in that study were applied to the consortium's educational partnership model as it gathered evaluations from field and academic faculties, planners, students, and graduates. Evaluation results contributed to improved educational content. Several publications in the compilation address the issue of social work in health care as a specialization and reflect the author bios for a social-health care concentration in the schools of social work.

A number of articles address the development of leadership skills. The division and the department of social work services established a leadership training exchange program, initiated in 1988 with Israeli social workers in health care settings and expanded in 1990 to include Australian social workers. The exchange program was designed to "enhance leadership capabilities, enrich . . . knowledge and skills needed to implement quality program . . . help assess current programs, contribute to their improvement and draw on and conduct applied studies to generate relevant information in order to offer recommendations for social-health policy with the ability to translate to cost-effective service programs." The program has demonstrated that participants can develop leadership capabilities when the learning/teaching curriculum is based on the expressed needs of experienced social work managers. Those who participated shared comparable philosophy and mission, services, fiscal concerns, staff structures, and practice settings. These similarities as well as national and cultural differences established the basis for a dynamic international educational exchange. Compelling evidence to date indicates that such a global exchange of social workers can be productive and successful.

EDUCATION OF OTHER HEALTH CARE PROFESSIONALS

THE CHALLENGE

Since its early beginnings in medical settings and in mental health programs, social work has both contributed to and been influenced by sociology, medicine, and psychiatry. In its earlier form, social work brought a social-environmental component to medical and psychiatric diagnosis and treatment formulations. Over time, a biopsychosocial frame of reference was developed as the philosophical basis of patient care, and social work participated in this formulation as well.

THE RELEVANT LITERATURE

Social workers have long recognized that collaboration with other health care professionals is critical to effective inpatient care and to successful community outreach. The development of a school of medicine in the mid-1960s added medical education to the institutional mission and expanded its research enterprise. Community health needs elicited the creation of a department of community medicine, which has been comprised of a multiprofessional faculty designed to educate medical students to practice in a social-health environment. To help achieve that objective a division of social work was established in community medicine. From the outset, social workers served as faculty in partnership with other disciplines in community medicine to develop a biopsychosocial and environmental framework (Bosch & Deuschle, 1989).

Social work faculty members, clinicians, and administrators alike contribute to the curriculum in areas of human growth and development; psychosocial functioning of individuals and groups; the impact of social needs, social and environmental circumstances, and social provisions and deficits on the development of illness; and the maintenance of health and the delivery of medical and social-health care services.

The social work clinical staff and faculty participate in required and elective educational programs of the medical school, providing teaching and learning opportunities for medical students, social work students, and students from other health care professions. The curriculum includes:

- the effect of social needs and the personal condition on health status and their effect on access to services;
- societal provisions for the promotion and maintenance of health, and the prevention of disease;
- patterns in health care planning, policy development, financing and the organization of services;
- the emergence of consumer concerns in securing a place in health care;
- quality improvement and professional accountability;
- a social-health frame of reference to all aspects of health care;
- an epidemiologic approach to understanding persons-at-risk.
- the place of the family in the support and care of individuals;
- the place of community social services in the support and care of those in need;
- the impact of the complex health organization on patient care;
- the partnership between patients and providers; and
- interprofessional service delivery as a tenet in social-health care.

Social work assumes a major role in medical education in the medical school. It participates in determining educational policies and practices, in developing curriculum, and in determining social work content in the implementation of objectives, the instruction of medical students in a wide range of experiences, graduate education through internship and residency programs, and continuing education of practicing health care professionals. Social work collaborates in research with a wide range of medical departments and plays a key role in a partnership with the community in the planning and delivery of community-based services. Clinicians, who might also be faculty members, carry out these functions in their practice or in their specific teaching responsibilities in medical education.

The published writings address social workers' roles in medical education, framed by their investment in community medicine. One article describes collaboration between social workers and their health care colleagues to develop an introduction to medicine course for beginning medical students. And social work practitioners were key to facilitating a community medicine clerkship that introduced students to the patient experience, including the impact of the illness, the home setting, and the community agency investment in care.

Another article addresses the community medicine clerkship and the impact of a multiprofessional faculty on student understanding of illness and available resources. Social work faculty members serve as tutors in the four-week community medicine clerkship required for third-year medical students. A social worker has co-directed the course for more than a decade. The goal of the rotation is to help medical students define and analyze a population-based medical problem. Working alone or in pairs, students select a community medicine topic and define a specific research question germane to that topic. They review the literature, choose a research design, gather and analyze data, interpret the data, and draw conclusions and recommendations. Social work tutors guide them through the clerkship requirements.

Another article addresses an interdisciplinary curriculum that trains medical students to work with terminally ill children and their families. Social workers teach content and interviewing skills in a curriculum component that addresses the impact of illness on patients and families.

Collaborative relationships among multiprofessional health team educators are not without their differences and tensions. One article describes the problems and benefits of team teaching of medical students. Another, written in 1968, is visionary in its description of trends and issues in interprofessional education. In citing the need for collaboration among professionals, the authors suggest that medical and social work students do not have "to think alike" but need to learn "to act together" to achieve collaboration in social-health care.

A series of articles describes educational activities related to services for the elderly. When geriatrics was introduced into the institution both as a medical division and department, social workers developed health education content that addressed a number of important issues, including sexuality in older persons, expanding lay education about diseases such as cancer and prostate disorders, and detecting elder abuse. They also developed a rationale to identify the issues and suggest intervention strategies. When geriatrics developed into a major primary care program, social workers assumed teaching and consultative roles to medical residents. Social workers joined in creating a geriatric team to provide inpatient education and consultation to practitioners. Social workers taught nurses' aides how to work with elderly Alzheimer patients, and they created a nurses' support group to help address nurses' concerns and feelings about the impact of AIDs.

CONCLUSION

Social work achievements in continuing education, in student education, and in the education of other health professionals support the premise that practice and programs must be of good quality and must be provided in valued settings to ensure sound education. But social work cannot rest on its laurels. It is in a vulnerable position not only in service delivery but also in education. Because its scope encompasses management, program development, community networking, and new functions and roles wherever clientele in need are found, education for social work practice must expand beyond its present boundaries. The skills social workers have today may not suffice for tomorrow in this cost-conscious health care environment. The current system for the education of social workers may not be adequate for the skills required in the coming decade (Christ, 1996). In addition to teaching the behavioral and social sciences, it may be essential to educate social workers to:

- understand organizational dynamics, the constraints and the translation of policy to program (services), focusing on the individual and the family;
- deliver social work care in primary care practices and community-based settings, rather than solely in hospitals;
- implement a more advanced practice as self-directed, independent workers;
- draw on consultation from social work and other disciplinary expertise;
- work in a wide range of financially maintained programs (e.g., managed care, HMOs, fee-for-service, group practice);

- develop collaborative skills for a multiprofessional practice and program planning;
- self-evaluate practice and services; be outcome-focused with the ability to draw conclusions for change as necessary; assume professional accountability;
- participate in education of social work students and in educational programs for other health care professionals;
- recruit and retrain minority social workers and those who wish to advance in the field;
- collaborate with academic social work;
- understand the value of information and its utilization;
- design and participate in applied studies;
- assist in better distribution of social work services in underserved and rural areas;
- enhance skills in short-term goal-focused treatment, with rapid assessment skills;
- participate in community-based activities; be aware of community wants and relevant data;
- listen to the consumer's voice for service delivery and needs;
- participate actively in outreach programs;
- educate the public about what to expect from a health care system and how to use it;
- educate the public about self-care and health maintenance;
- participate actively in small group education regarding disease prevention;
- learn the benefits of a professional role in a collaborative practice;
- obtain continuing education about diseases and their consequences, with emphasis on social and physical functional limitations;
- develop a major concentration on the elderly, the disabled, the vulnerable, and other major users of health care;
- develop greater awareness of social illnesses;
- define the role of social workers in service and in social action; and
- enter into coalitions to enhance the social-health of the community.

Market forces affect schools of social work and health care organizations. Each has responded to these forces in different ways. Downsizing, reengineering of service delivery and staffing, and the impact of managed care payment services have affected the educational and research commitments of academic medical centers. Teaching hospitals have a history of educating future health care professionals and developing innovative care through their research endeavors. The funding sources for support of professional education and study must continue to safeguard the quality of health care. Health care agencies need schools of social work and schools need health agencies. We must create a set of educational processes through which schools; the field; students; other health care professionals, including public health practitioners; payers; and clients forge a new set of relationships that provide social work a bridge to the new world of health care and social services.

Educating for social work practice in health care requires a consortium of the many parties involved in health services to create a curriculum and practice for today and tomorrow. The complementary structure would allow for joint deliberation, decision making, and appropriate practice in:

- giving practice representation in curriculum development and in educational goal determination;
- making available a reservoir of resources in the field where innovative programs are underway, or where new ideas could be tested by bringing the school into the field beyond the immediate student need;
- making available the opportunity to teach appropriate concepts and theory in the appropriate locus (i.e., to broaden the concept of the campus, include the agency setting, and relate to the realities of a complex multiprofessional system);
- making available a wider range of agency programs and activities including a range of processes and functions as learning opportunities;
- offering continuing education opportunities developed in joint deliberations;
- permitting an exchange of staff between school and practice, in a lend-lease sabbatical or planned arrangement on agreed-upon objectives, such as to teach a session, a course, develop staff, and so forth, allowing for valid financial and university and agency support mechanisms, and to remain current with practice and education;
- developing a set of guidelines and expectations for experiential learning, shared with students and made a conscious component of curriculum;
- developing standards for instructional centers and field education, with recognition through awards of faculty rank;
- making research principles, methodology, and applied studies a conscious process by the joint development of: a) measurements for the effectiveness of education; b) assessment methods of social ser-

vices, utilization patterns, allocation, effectiveness, quality, and cost allocation, with particular emphasis on professional accountability; c) assessment methods of utilization of differential manpower; and d) assessment methods of studies to enhance knowledge and skills and for the implementation of program change;

- making overt the cost of all aspects of the educational expectations and jointly seeking support; and

- making available to lay groups the understanding and knowledge relevant to achieving the common goal, enlisting appropriate lay representation in the deliberations (Rehr & Rosenberg, 1977; pp. 247–248)

MOUNT SINAI REFERENCES

EDUCATING FOR SOCIAL-HEALTH CARE: SOCIAL WORK PRACTITIONERS, STUDENTS AND OTHER HEALTH CARE PROFESSIONALS

1950s

Siegel D (1959). Supervision in social work. In MHP Finn, F Brown (Eds.). *Training in Clinical Psychology*. New York: International University Press:86–94.

1960s

Dana B, Sheps C (1968). Trends and issues in interprofessional education: Pride, prejudice and progress. *Education for Social Work*, Fall:35–41.
Rehr H (1962). *An experiment in evolving an integrated staff development program*. Monograph. New York: The United Hospital Fund, June.
White E (1961). The role of the community in rehabilitation. *Social Casework*, July.

1970s

Aufses A, Dana B (1972). Introduction to medicine: A developmental history and analysis of an interdepartmental course. In VW Lippard, E Purcell (Eds.). *The Changing Medical Curriculum—Report of a Macy Conference*. New York: Josiah Macy, Jr. Foundation.
Banta D, Jackson G, Dana B, Bosch SJ, Mulvihill M (1976). Teaching community medicine by clerkship. *Academic Relationships and Teaching Resources*. Washington DC: Government Printing Office, 7:101–106.
Berkman B (1978). *Knowledge Base and Program Needs for Effective Social Work Practice in Health: A Review of the Literature*. Monograph. Society for Hospital Social Work Directors. Chicago, IL: American Hospital Association.
Caroff P, Wilson M (1979). Social work education for professional accountability: The Hunter College School of Social Work and Mount Sinai School of Medicine consortium. In H Rehr (Ed.). *Professional Accountability for Social Work Practice: A Search for Concepts and Guidelines*. New York: Prodist:128–141.

Deuschle K, Bosch S, Banta HD, Dana B (1972). The community medicine clerk-ship: A learner-centered program. *Journal of Medical Education*, 47:931–938.

Reinherz H, Berkman B, Grob M, Ewalt P (1977). Training in accountability: A social work mandate. *Health and Social Work*, 2(2):43.

Regensburg J (1979). *Toward Education for Health Professions*. New York: Harper & Row.

Rosenberg G, Brenner B (1978). Self-directed social workers: Continuing education in the health care setting. *Quality Review Bulletin*, March:18–19.

Rosenberg G (1979). Continuing education and the self-directed worker.In H Rehr (Ed.). *Professional Accountability for Social Work Practice: A Search for Concepts and Guidelines*. New York: Prodist:111–127.

Toller R, Amorosa K, Garfield M (1980). Notes from the field: The development of a teaching tool. In P Caroff, MD Mailick (Eds). *An Academic-Practice Partnership*. New York:Prodist:97–105.

Young AT (1979). The chart notation. In H Rehr (Ed.). *Professional Accountability for Social Work Practice: A Search for Concepts and Guidelines*. New York: Prodist: 62–73.

1980s

Bennett C, Grob G (1982). The social worker new to health care: Basic learning tasks. *Social Work in Health Care*, 8(2):49–64.

Bennett C, Beckerman N (1986). The drama of discharge: Worker/supervisor perspectives. *Social Work in Health Care*,11(3):1–12.

Bennett C, Blumenfield S (1989). Enhancing social work practice in health care: A deeper look at behavior in the work place. *The Clinical Supervisor*, 7(2/3):71–88.

Bloom J, Ansell P, Bloom M (1989). Detecting elder abuse: A guide for physicians. *Geriatrics*, 44(6):40–44,56.

Blumenfield S, Morrison B, Stroh J, Fizdale R (1981). The elderly and the social health care continuum. *Mount Sinai Journal of Medicine*, 48(6):569–572.

Blumenfield S, Morris J, Sherman FT (1982). The geriatric team in the acute care hospital: An educational and consultation modality. *Journal of the American Geriatrics Society*, 30(10):660–664.

Blumenfield S (1983). A summer fellowship program in gerontological social work in health care. *Journal of Gerontological Social Work*, 5(3):61–75.

Blumenfield S (1985). Gerontology journal club: A continuing education modality for experienced social workers in an acute hospital setting. *The Gerontologist*, 25(1):11–14.

Butler R, Lewis M (1981). Aging and sexuality. *Journal of the Western Gerontological Society*, Fall:5,41.

Caroff P, Rehr H (1985). The Hunter-Mount Sinai social work consortium: History, objectives and roles. In P Caroff, H Rehr (Eds.). *A New Model in an Academic-Practice Partnership*. Lexington, MA: Ginn Press:1–9.

Chan JM, Cincotta N (1981). Training students to work with terminally ill children in a child life program. In R Debellis (Ed.). *The Housestaff and Thanatology*. Salem, NH:Arno Press:111–117.

Cincotta N (1983). Commentary on Neil Bracht's 'preparing new generations of social workers for practice in health settings.' In G Rosenberg, H Rehr (Eds.). *Advancing Social Work Practice in the Health Care Field*. New York:Haworth Press: 48–51.

Clarke S, Neuwirth L, Bernstein R (1986). An expanded social work role in a university hospital-based group practice: Service provider, physician educator and organizational consultant. *Social Work in Health Care,* 11(4):1–18.

Cloward L (1983). Commentary on Bess Dana's 'the social work-community medicine connection.' *Social Work in Health Care,* 8(3):25–27.

Dana B (1983). The social work-community medicine connection. *Social Work in Health Care,* 8(3):11–23.

Dana B (1985). The educational challenge. In H Rehr, P Caroff (Eds.). *A New Model in an Academic-Practice Partnership.* Lexington, MA: Ginn Press:65–70.

Furman L, Walther V, Wilson M (1980). Developing an educational team in a complex hospital setting. In P Caroff, MD Mailick (Eds.). *Social Work in Health Services: An Academic-Practice Partnership.* New York:Prodist:87–96.

Gantt A, Hopkins M, Pinsky S, Tuzman L (1989). The training of social work students in the psychoeducation model of family treatment. *Journal of Teaching in Social Work,* 3(1):35–43.

Gladstein M, Wilson M (1980). Three field teaching centers in the social health module. In P Caroff, MD Mailick (Eds.). *Social Work in Health Services: An Academic-Practice Partnership.* New York: Prodist:65–86.

Gordon N (1982). *Organizational change in a medical setting: A field work curriculum for direct practice students.* Dissertation. City University of New York, June.

Hunsdon S, Clarke S (1984). The impact of illness on patients and families: Social workers teach medical students. *Social Work in Health Care,*10(2):41–52.

Lewis M, Osako M (1985). Conversation with a geisha. *Quarante: Magazine for the Woman Who's Arrived,* 33–39.

Lowe JI (1985). The practice teaching dyad: A preceptor's view. In H Rehr, P Caroff (Eds.). *A New Model in an Academic-Practice Partnership.* Lexington, MA: Ginn Press:29–34.

Lurie A, Rosenberg G (Eds.) (1984). *Social Work Administration in Health Care.* New York: Haworth Press.

Mailick M (1985). Developing the academic component. In H Rehr, P Caroff (Eds.). *A New Model in an Academic-Practice Partnership.* Lexington, MA: Ginn Press: 11–18.

Morrison B (1980). Commentary on Rosalie Kane's 'knowledge development for social work practice in health.' *Social Work in Health Care,* 8(3):73–76.

Morrison B, Rehr H (1985). Evaluating the consortium: Planners, faculty, preceptors, and graduates. In H Rehr, P Caroff (Eds.). *A New Model in an Academic-Practice Partnership.* Lexington, MA: Ginn Press:39–64.

Reardon GT (1987). *Control of Deviant Behavior in a Psychiatric Hospital.* Dissertation. Rutgers, The State University of New Jersey.

Rehr H, Berkman B, Rosenberg G (1980). A new approach to appraising student field experiences in health settings. In P Caroff, M Mailick (Eds.). *Social Work in Health Services: An Academic-Practice Partnership.* New York: Prodist:131–153.

Rehr H, Rosenberg G (1984). Today's education for today's health care social work practice. In A Lurie, G Rosenberg (Eds.). *Social Work Administration in Health Care.* New York: Haworth Press:99–108. Also in *Clinical Social Work Journal* (1977), 5(4):342–350.

Rehr H, Caroff P (1985). *A New Model in an Academic-Practice Partnership: Multi-Instructor and Institutional Collaboration.* Lexington, MA: Ginn Press.

Rehr H, Caroff P, Wilson M (1985). The participants deliberate. In H Rehr, P Caroff (Eds.). *A New Model in an Academic-Practice Partnership.* Lexington, MA: Ginn Press:71–79.

Rehr H, Caroff P (1985). Conclusions and recommendations. In H Rehr, P Caroff (Eds.). *A New Model in an Academic-Practice Partnership.* Lexington, MA: Ginn Press:81–89.

Rehr H, Brown M, Corry JM, Murray R, Elster SK (1984). Case study: Mount Sinai School of Medicine. In SJ Brody, NA Persily (Eds.). *Hospitals and the Aged.* Rockville, MD: Aspen Press:237–245.

Richardson J (1985). The practice teaching dyad: A graduate student's view. In H Rehr, P Caroff (Eds.). *A New Model in an Academic-Practice Partnership.* Lexington, MA: Ginn Press:34–37.

Rosenberg G, Rehr H (Eds.) (1983). *Advancing Social Work Practice in the Health Care Field: Emerging Issues and New Perspectives.* New York: Haworth Press.

Rosenberg G (1986). Social work in the future: Predictions and strategies. *Current Issues in Health Care for Professional Leaders: Problems and Potentials and Changes in Health Care: A Challenge to the Profession.* Monograph. New York: Mount Sinai Medical Center:(May):35–46.

Shein L (1983). Commentary on Bess Dana's 'the social work-community medicine connection.' In G Rosenberg H Rehr (Eds.). *Social Work in Health Care, 8*(3): 23–24.

Showers N (1988). *Factors Associated with Graduate Social Work Student Satisfaction in Hospital Field Education Programs.* Dissertation. City University of New York, 1–317.

Siegel ME (1987). Psychosocial Aspects of Chemotherapy in Cancer Care: The Patient, Family and Staff. In R Debellis, G Hyman, A Kutscher, ME Siegel (Eds.). New York: Haworth Press.

Silverton M (1983). Commentary on Rosalie Kane's 'knowledge development for social work practice in health.' *Social Work in Health Care, 8*(3):70–73.

Simon EP (1988). Integrating research and practice in the workplace. *Social Work Research and Abstracts,* Summer:4–5.

Speedling E, McDermott M, Eichhorn S, Rosenberg G (1987). Hospital employee-patient relations: A program for enhancing patient well-being. *Hospital and Health Services Administration,* February:71–82.

Stein E, Wade K, Smith D (1991). Clinical support groups that work. *Journal of the Association of Nurses in AIDS Care, 2*:29–36.

Toller R, Amorose K, Garfield M (1980). Notes from the field: The development of a teaching tool. In P Caroff, MD Mailick (Eds.). *Social Work in Health Services: An Academic-Practice Partnership.* New York: Prodist:97–108.

Wilson M (1985). Developing the practice component. In H Rehr, P Caroff (Eds.). *A New Model in an Academic-Practice Partnership.* Lexington, MA: Ginn Press:19–27.

Young AT (1983). Commentary on Neil Bracht's 'preparing new generations of social workers for practice in health settings.' In G Rosenberg, H Rehr (Eds.). *Advancing Social Work Practice in the Health Care Field.* New York: Haworth Press:51–54.

1990s

Bernstein SR (1991). Contracted services: Issues for the non-profit agency manager. *Sector Quality, 22*:429–443.

Bernstein SR (1991). *Managing Contracted Services in the Non-profit Agency: Administrative Ethical and Political Issues*. Philadelphia, PA: Temple University Press.

Blumenfield S, Simon EP, Bennett C (1991). The legal clinic: Helping social workers master the legal environment in health care. *Social Work in Health Care, 16*(2): 7–19.

Cincotta N, Levine E, McClean K (1990). *Radiotherapy Days*. Monograph. New York: Mount Sinai Medical Center.

Gantt A, Pinsky S, Rock B, Rosenberg E (1990). Practice research center: A field/class model to teach research, practice and values. In D Schneck (Ed.). *Field Education in Social Work*. Dubuque, IA: Kendall-Hunt.

Gantt A, Pinsky S, Rock B, Rosenberg E (1990). Practice and research: An integrative approach. *Journal of Teaching in Social Work, 4*(1):129–143.

Mailick MD (1991). Editorial: Recruitment and MSW graduates. *Social Work in Health Care*,16–14.

Rehr H (1991). An academic practice partnership in social work education. In C Irizarry, C James (Eds.). *Achieving Excellence in Health Social Work*. Adelaide, Australia: Flinders Press:85–96.

Rosengarten L, Smith G (1990). Training aides in caring for persons with dementia. *Pride Institute Journal of Long-Term Home Health Care, 9*:56–59.

Showers N (1990). Hospital graduate social work field work programs: A study in New York City. *Health and Social Work, 15*(1):55–63.

Showers N, Cuzzi L (1991). What field instructors of social work students need from hospital field work programs. *Social Work in Health Care*,16(1):39–52.

Siegel ME (1990). Rites of passage/rights of passage. In A Kutscher, S Bess, S Klagsbrun, ME Siegel, DJ Cherico, L Kutscher, D Peretz, FE Selder (Eds.). *For the Bereaved: The Road to Recovery*. Philadelphia, PA: Charles Press.

Silberman JM (1991). The AIDS epidemic: Professional and personal concerns of graduate social work students in field placement. *Social Work in Health Care, 15*(3):77–100.

Silver A, Schechter C, Walther V, Deuschle K (1991). Development of faculty consultants in a problem-based third year community medicine clerkship. *Journal of Community Health, 16*(3):133–141.

11

A Prescription for Social-Health Care: Responding to the Client, the Community, and the Organization

Helen Rehr, Gary Rosenberg, and Susan Blumenfield

THE CHANGING FACE OF HEALTH CARE

For more than a century, controversy has existed about the provision of medical care in this country. From its barbershop beginnings before the Flexner report and the early projections of Theodore Roosevelt's 1912 health campaign rhetoric for "the adoption of a system of social insurance" to this last decade of the 20th century, medical care has been a public health issue that has either loomed large or been dormant in the political arena. As we near the end of this century, health care is in crisis, the industry in turmoil. The fiscal crisis and financial reimbursement programs are dictating major changes and are shifting health care delivery from the concept of a social utility to privatization under a number of systems. The public has inadequate knowledge of the changing patterns; individuals respond to systems of care based on needs. A national social-health policy does not exist. Millions of the country's people have no, or limited, access to medical care.

Most people agree that almost 20 years of cost containment, competition, regulation, and deregulation have barely controlled the financial hemorrhaging in a system that may be the world's most sophisticated, but that costs too much and does not serve everyone. How to safeguard access to care while cutting costs is a goal that continues to elude politicians. As health care costs continue to escalate, so too does consensus about the need for major change in the system. Congressional committees are charged with finding solutions to the rate of increase in patient and payer expenses.

They seek ways to change the U.S. health care system, making it fiscally viable while ensuring access and quality. But it is doubtful that a sound federal social-health policy will be forthcoming in the near future.

The predominant values that influence today's health care delivery system are private market decision making and shared responsibility. In earlier times, shared responsibility meant that the government and the voluntary sector were jointly responsive to local residents and their community needs. Today it refers to the joint responsibility of the individual consumer and third-party payers. Market-based decision making is eroding certain principles of voluntary and government-sponsored health care.

Medical institutions are adopting organizational approaches borrowed from industry. In so doing, some hope to survive on their own. Others affiliate, merge with, or buy other institutions. Some join together to self-insure their services. Still others limit care to patients or to their communities based on how they are paid. The charitable view held by voluntary nonprofit organizations in response to local needs (the Hill-Burton principle) is being lost. However, the medical institutions that still see the benefits of upholding their mission to serve their communities are forming coalitions, combining services, and preserving a partnership with their communities.

The 1990 estimated costs of health care were 12.2% of GNP, distributed as follows: private, 33%; Medicare, 20%; out-of-pocket, 17%; state and local, 13%; Medicaid, 11%; other private, 5%. Although private insurance, out-of-pocket, and other private sources totaled 55% for that period, the accelerating costs of care continue to have an impact on all payers. The question now being raised is not only what to cut, but how extensive the cutbacks should be and how to contain future costs.

MANAGED CARE AS THE SOLUTION

The concept of managed care was touted as the life raft for the traditional health care industry, which is costly and sinking. Managed care is a method of coordinating and delivering health care through a range of provider networks such as the traditional health maintenance organization (HMO), a preferred provider organization (PPO), a point-of-service (POS) contract, or a self-insured managed-care (SIMC) system. These programs operate with primary care physicians who provide most services and screen referrals to other providers. Although managed-care programs have proliferated, they are still untested in terms of performance, quality of care, efficiency, or commitment to low-income patients, those with complex illnesses, physician autonomy, and the certification of other social and health care providers.

PREVENTION AND PRIMARY CARE

Prevention and primary care are two important components in managed care. The premise of prevention is to keep managed care beneficiaries healthy and out of medical care and thus yield savings in future health care costs. For those with acute illnesses, a predictable course of treatment, and no unusual consequences, managed care, assuming quality, should be good. But when specialized and ongoing care is essential, as for those with chronic illnesses, obstacles to needed services may arise. Financial considerations appear to influence medical decision making, set by benefit coverage imposed by institutional plans.

The increased managed care penetration into health care has made its delivery more competitive in business terms. It functions to monitor and to authorize the use of health services by drawing on negotiated payment methods and utilization controls. The plans do not guarantee access to care, and their rules and regulations can obstruct an individual's use of services. By seeking low-cost providers willing to follow guidelines and control access, managed care insurers have proved profitable enterprises.

REVIEWS OF MANAGED CARE PROGRAMS

A review of managed care in Los Angeles found lower hospital costs, reduced lengths-of-stay, and decreased morbidity rates in contrast to health care markets with little managed care. The study suggests that managed care "may have a positive impact on patient care" (Currents, June 20, 1995; p. 12).

A recent review of managed care plans, funded by the Commonwealth Fund, found a number of concerns and some positive aspects. On the one hand, the review identified practices that encouraged underutilization, ineffective quality standards and monitoring, reduced payment levels to providers, barriers to specialized services, and obstacles in addressing consumer complaints. On the other hand, it identified reduced administrative costs, reduced emergency room use, support of primary care, and enhanced control and coordination of care. The programs, however, lacked orientation and education of enrollees, support systems for patients in need, and mechanisms to address provider or consumer questions. They also lacked provisions to address the uninsured or those who had lost coverage, and regulation of products did not occur (Davis, 1996).

As managed care plans increase in number, competition will be the driving factor in health care delivery, with a growing emphasis on developing primary care physicians as gatekeepers to services and a decrease in enrollees in medical schools. Inpatient utilization will continue to decline, and hospital beds will close in deference to ambulatory care arrangements. Mergers will occur as institutions and providers align programs and enhance market share, while strengthening their positions to negotiate reimbursement rates with payers or to self-insure.

IMPACT ON ACADEMIC CENTERS

Not-for-profit institutions, particularly university hospitals and their faculties, are feeling the impact of these changes on their programs as private insurers limit what they will reimburse. These academic centers represent 6% (300) of hospitals in the country, but account for 20% (one in five) of inpatient admissions and are dominant in urban centers (*Hospitals*, January 1996; p. 22). As teaching medical institutions, many have commitments to their local communities to provide services. They give a considerable portion of limited payment and uncompensated services to the poor in blighted urban areas. They are focused largely on inpatient services, which are their primary revenue base.

In the past 15 years, hospital admissions have plummeted, and health care dollars are shifting to ambulatory arenas. Although the academic centers deliver emergency and acute care, they are largely specialized and just beginning to develop resources for primary care. They face competition from other providers outside the institutions, such as freestanding facilities. As they face reimbursement limits, academic institutions are attempting to create arrangements that will ensure their survival. To be competitive, they are forming self-insured and capitation group practices for employees, medical staff clientele, and Medicare and Medicaid recipients.

FOUR-TIER SYSTEM OF CARE

Without a national health policy, the future delivery of health care might well be based on a four-tier payment system. In such a system, Tier 1 might be a private fee-for-service system for the wealthy; Tier 2, employee-employer managed care for the majority of workers and families under a shared insurance premium and co-payment program; Tier 3, government-funded managed care programs for the elderly, disabled, and selected populations; and Tier 4, state-governed managed care for the poor and uninsured, a state-dominated type of Medicaid managed care. Most likely, Medicaid programs would be covered by block grants to states, perhaps with some federal guidelines. In the 4-tier system, health care services would take place in hospitals that are more commercial than voluntary in their administration, and in government-operated institutions such as the Veteran's Administration, domiciliary or residential facilities for the mentally or developmentally disabled, and municipal hospitals. However, if New York City is an example, a trend toward privatization of municipal hospitals is in the offing.

The major change will be in the shift from inpatient to ambulatory care programs, which will include group HMO-type practices, solo practices (fast disappearing), clinics, neighborhood primary care centers, emergency centers, and a range of specialized services such as sports medicine, women's health, and geriatric centers, either commercially owned or under the aegis of medical institutions.

As a trend develops toward larger and more complex integrated health care organizations with decreased emphasis on inpatient care (bed capacity is controlled), we see hospitalization reserved for sicker patients who need specialized and/or technological care. The majority of services already have shifted to ambulatory care programs that include the fast-growing, one-day surgical and technological interventions.

PROFESSIONAL TURMOIL

Payment approaches have thrown the health care professions into turmoil. Tensions have developed among physician groups and among other health care disciplines. Boundaries have become fuzzy as competition and turf battles incur instability. A proliferation of nonmedical personnel is occurring in the counseling, support, and fringe health services. These new providers create an expanding health care industry of nonsupervised and nonregulated enterprises that run the gamut of alternative therapeutic programs. Self-help groups also are proliferating for alcoholism, substance abuse, person abuse, disease-specific categories, and bereavement. Overwhelming in number, they often operate without professional guidance.

In addition, advances in medical technology continue to occur. Many are costly miracles, such as heart transplants for the very few. New biomedical knowledge should bring new awareness and knowledge about one's physical and personal self. Such knowledge should result in more self-care, health maintenance, and a learned means to a quality life style.

However, sound self-care requires an educated and motivated public prepared to be responsive to its own health maintenance.

SOCIAL-HEALTH PROBLEMS
AND SOCIAL WORK SERVICES

People's behaviors and their areas of interest can reflect the societal patterns of the times, culture, and/or the concerns of a region or a locale. Social ills and illnesses exist that command ongoing professional commitment. Despite many public health gains, social-health problems have proliferated, some of the most severe being:

- inequities in health services; barriers to access affect millions of uninsured and underinsured;
- problems of poverty, homelessness, and hunger that undermine individual health;
- excessive behaviors; social disorders reaching near epidemic proportions, including person abuse, violence, accidents, suicides, drug and substance abuse;
- social diseases resulting from life style, environmental and work conditions, including AIDS, cirrhosis, emphysema, coronary disorders;
- uninsured persons who seek medical care late, arrive with advanced illness, and misuse emergency services;
- sicker patients with multiple and severe chronic illnesses making greater demands on hospitals and their staffs;
- lack of preventive and health maintenance services;
- limited and costly at-home care resources in the community;
- the growing numbers of individuals who seek care for stress, fear, and anxiety arising out of stressful daily living patterns and occupational "hazards;"
- those with social-psychological disorders evidenced in both physical and mental health symptoms;
- the growing numbers of physically disabled and handicapped person; and
- the increasing numbers of developmentally disabled persons.

These are the social-health problems that people present in vast numbers to medical institutions and providers. For most social ailments and diseases, medical care has been the primary means to relieve symptoms.

That care, however, frequently is fragmented, neither coordinated nor comprehensive, often indicative of overuse, underuse, and/or misuse induced by either an individual or provider.

The underlying factors that drive an individual to excess require a more focused social-health approach. Such an approach includes "counseling, support services, and health education leading to self-care and to motivation to change existing life style patterns" (Miller & Rehr, 1983; p. 258). The social-environmental ills affecting large numbers of the population require deliberation among multiple professional disciplines, consumers, and business and government, to arrive at a sound social-health policy and the resources to implement it.

Social and political events have affected the place of social work in the domain of service to people. In viewing just the past 50 years, one recognizes the impact of World War II as social work gained status in the military, in selective service, in world-based organizations such as the Red Cross at the end of the war, and in key positions in veterans' programs. Post-World War II, a time of general affluence, gave rise to one of the most progressive periods for government programs in U.S. history and social-health programs proliferated.

The federal government advanced social work's status in health care via legislation in the 1960s. It endorsed medical social services to recipients of government-supported health services for military personnel and selected beneficiaries of Medicare, Medicaid, and maternal and child health services. But although social work in health care gained some prominence, it never gained power. Its roles in health care, given the biomedical model, were largely incremental. Social workers worked beside medicine in a medical model of care that was individual/patient-focused.

The medical institution, under the joint aegis of medical and lay leaders, essentially is dominated by physicians. In the past 50 years, social work has striven to bring a biopsychosocial focus into medical care by demonstrating the impact of social and environmental factors on patient and family attitudes and behaviors and on diagnosis, treatment, compliance, and self-care. As medicine came to value the biopsychosocial components, physicians and their institutions moved from a disease-and-disorder view of medicine to a more comprehensive social-health approach to care.

As incremental changes in health care philosophy and delivery occurred, social work found itself in a collaborative partnership with other health care professionals, while at the same time it had begun to seek autonomy with the right to regulate and control its own activities. It emphasized a knowledge base and values and skills, sought licensing and accreditation, supported an association, and controlled education for the field (Kerson, 1981; p. 159). It sought professional status on a par with other health care professionals. Progress was evidenced in medicine and social work. The health care field had gained tremendously in what it had to offer individuals in managing disease, disorders, and disabilities. In spite of economic waves in the nation, the medical establishment developed more innovations in these 50 years than in all its history. But, the tide began to turn in the 1970s when the country suffered a short recession. It accelerated in the 1980s when social events, social problems, and a fiscal crisis fostered a general conservatism that resulted in the election of a conservative government. Deregulation, privatization, and corporate supremacy became the vogue. An overspent government gave industry the leeway to privatize much of the health care system, shifting it away from a voluntary, public health social utility.

Today, economic changes, with their impact on industry, government, charities, and individual life styles, have again produced uncertainty and even conflict among disciplines. Currently, only a tenuous cooperation exists among them, as all aspects of the health care field have been and are continuing to be threatened by severe cutbacks and reorganization in the patterns of health care delivery.

Survival is today's major concern. Although social work has found a key place in health care in spite of waves of crises, it must find ways to hold and enhance its position. The rationale for social work services in health settings is set by a number of assumptions:

- A biopsychosocial focus is required to deal with the needs of individuals who are sick and disabled.
- A multiprofessional program that recognizes biopsychosocial factors in the care of individuals, and the scope of their cultural diversity is essential to quality care.
- A working partnership between professionals and the consumers of their care is essential for informed decision making.
- Services should be accessible, available, and affordable to all in need.
- Services should be comprehensive, coordinated, and continuous to allow individuals to achieve maximum benefits.
- Prescribed opportunities to assess and reassess programs should exist.
- Changes projected from evaluations should be understood and implemented by staff affected.
- Shared professional and consumer responsibility for planning and implementing necessary health care services is essential to affect the health status of the community and public social-health policy.

The assumptions support the premise that care of the sick and the infirm and prevention of illness require a social-health formulation, an example of which, offered by Kotelchuck (1992), calls for a health care system in balance (see Figure 11.1). It also calls for roles and functions for social work in health care even as health care is changing. Social work has made many contributions and more must be projected for the future. Social work has thus far played an important role in:

- the acute care of patients, setting in motion quality discharge planning with counseling and resource information, affecting length of stay;
- primary care, providing psychosocial assessments for integrated care and facilitating patients' access to needed community services;
- counseling patients and supporting family members in response to illness and expectations; assisting with decision making (Berkman, 1996; p. 544);
- emergency care—responding by crisis intervention, triage, and referring patients to appropriate care sites; assisting in seeking entitlement benefits;
- assuring access to needed services by outreach and casefinding, eliminating obstacles to health promotion, maintenance, and prevention, by identifying those groups at high social-risk and by assisting in developing programs to support health education.

Health Education				Home Support Program
Health Promotion	Primary Care		Nursing Home Rehabilitation Assisted Living	
Community Partnership		Acute Care Tertiary Care Hospitals		

FIGURE 11.1.   Projecting a social-health model.

- long-term care and assistance in chronic illness, by social work treatment and investment in informal and formal support services within a design of continuous care;
- contributing to the development of a comprehensive and integrated social-health delivery system within medical institutions, and by serving as case managers to coordinate needed care;
- providing mental health counseling to those who are ill in both medical and psychiatric arenas;
- providing care within a patient-family focus; and
- providing consultation to other health care providers to address psychosocial and environmental needs.

The government's debt crisis became a paramount issue in the 1990s. Our legislators have moved to tackle the major social benefits designed for selected groups, and health services have been targeted and continue to be on the agenda for cutbacks. Social work services in health care is one of the targets. Across the country, programs have been downsized, eliminated, or reengineered into new service formats.

Why has social work been unable to find a permanent and more fundamental place in health care? It has been difficult to find voices for its services. Social work's objectives are to improve individual and family life and to mitigate social-health ills, at least in individuals it treats. Is the lack of public recognition and status because social work:

- is associated with the poor and needy, setting it in the welfare arena?
- labors with those who have little or no voice in society?
- works with physicians who still, despite their poor publicity, hold the reins and are chary of competition in health care?
- has not demonstrated to the public at-large its contributions?
- has not demonstrated cost-effective benefits to those served, nor to its other constituencies (e.g., payers, regulatory bodies).
- is expected by politicians to deal with multicausal social problems which require policy and program change and multidisciplinary investment?
- has not found a collaborative role with other health care professionals in addressing social-health issues?
- has been a charity and government-based supported service?
- has its own internecine battles—academics versus practitioners?

All of these issues have led to a general unease about the profession and uncertainty about its purpose and direction. The health and mental health care fields, which have had the largest numbers of social workers and have been responsible for the majority of counseling services, have not generally responded to questions that address their contributions.

SOCIAL-HEALTH CARE TODAY AND TOMORROW

As the end of the 20th century draws near, the state of health care is more uncertain than ever. The divisiveness among politicians, health care professionals, health care organizations, industry, insurance companies, and the public appears to preclude health care reform in the near future. Social commitment to health care access for all has steadily eroded. Many of the country's social programs are in jeopardy, as evidenced by the Congress's proposal to make substantial cuts in welfare, education, and health care which threaten to reverse the social gains of the past 60 years. Social-health problems in the United States continue to escalate. Limitations in service and access to care are serious obstacles to many individuals.

Economic imperatives are the driving force behind the radical change in health care and health care systems. The dramatic shift from an inpatient focus of care to an ambulatory care focus will continue to influence the shape of health care as institutions and medical professionals seek cost-effective alternatives to inpatient care, such as ambulatory surgery, same-day diagnostic consultations, redesigned clinics, and managed care group practices that provide laboratory, technological, and preventive services to their patients. In this environment, group practices will increase, community partnerships with the health care institutions will be essential, the architecture of the health care institution will change radically, the role of the government will shift, and the voice of the consumer will have to become much stronger.

GROUP PRACTICES

Physicians in group practices provide the majority of ambulatory care as the solo, fee-for-service practice has begun to disappear. Although fee-for-service reimbursement has not completely disappeared, group practices governed by managed-care reimbursement are more attractive to payer agencies. Group practice also is attractive to many physicians who perceive that working in a group is less demanding and more professionally supportive than working in a solo practice. They welcome the array of services offered by managed care group practices.

However, physicians are disturbed that managed care bureaucrats with no medical knowledge and no awareness of patient needs can disallow service reimbursement requests. Insurance companies appear to be setting institutional regulations not only for payment for services, but also for approval of care. As the number of programs grows, it will be essential to regulate insurers to guarantee access and availability of care and safeguard the doctor-patient partnership as well as the quality of care.

THE COMMUNITY

Medical institutions continue to respond to community needs. Institutional leaders are active in developing relationships, even partnerships, which ensure that local needs are understood and that address social-health needs. Urban-based medical institutions, located in blighted areas that house low-income and poverty-level families, encounter the effects of social-environmental blight on the health status of the disadvantaged. Blane (1995) suggests that "the distribution is not bipolar (the advantaged versus the rest) but graded, so that each change in the level of advantage or disadvantage is in general associated with a change in health" (p. 903). Health settings, particularly the urban voluntary medical institutions, have joined with neighbors and community social agencies in programs that benefit local residents.

Community medicine or public health departments in academic medical centers bring an epidemiological focus to identifying serious issues and vulnerable populations. Information is essential. Developing information about at-risk populations promotes more rational delivery of care. Regional health status indicators can inform the community and health providers about leading causes of disease and death. Information helps institutions further health promotion and planning with community residents.

Institutions that promote a community partnership open their doors to assure access. A number of regional medical institutions have grouped together to create a self-insurance managed care enterprise (SIMC) so they can contract with Medicaid for reimbursement. While organizing primary care for Medicaid patients, they also are introducing primary care to children and the elderly in organized group practices under their aegis. The SIMC plans probably will broaden to compete with the managed care plans of private insurance companies.

CHRONIC ILLNESS AND SOCIAL DISEASES

Chronic illnesses are primary health concerns in the United States. Although chronic illnesses usually have a physical or mental etiology, chronicity typically is accompanied by negative psychosocial and environmental factors. Chronic illness can affect role performance, response to therapy, dependence on people and equipment, social and daily living activities, and relationships with significant others. It also can affect the extent of hospitalization and nursing home admission, and ultimately one's death (Verbrugge & Patrick, 1995; p. 175).

Chronic conditions are found among all age groups and among both women and men, but the majority are found in the elderly who frequently suffer two or more comorbid chronic conditions. Although those with chronic illnesses make the greatest demand on medical services, Thomas (1977) notes that 75% of patient visits are those referred to as the worried well or the stabilized well and who seek help essentially because of stress, anxiety, depression, and fears (p. 42). Moreover, evidence exists that chronic disease and disability in the general public may be declining in the United States, largely because of changes in public hygiene, sanitation, nutrition, and life style. However, severity and disability in the old elderly with comorbid conditions remain critical.

In addition to long-term physical and emotional disorders, institutions face growing numbers of admissions of individuals with a range of social-health diseases and disorders. These are individuals engaged in behavioral excesses or exposed to detrimental social-environmental factors that can result in serious symptomatology. Many disorders occur as a result of self-imposed risks—such as excess alcohol, smoking, eating, and work. Careless living patterns can result in lung cancer, coronary and arterial diseases, ulcers, hypertension, obesity, cirrhosis, emphysema, and so forth. And accidents, violence, and abuse create the need for emergency services.

People seek help from medical sources for these disorders. Although medical care is needed, it will not mitigate underlying social-health problems that require motivation to change life style. Physicians are the least trained to deal with motivational drives. Counseling, support services, health promotion, and education are more successful methods to achieve change. But comprehensive care requires a team of skilled health care professionals who support health maintenance, based on studies of causation, individual life style, and understanding of biopsychosocial factors in socially based disorders.

SPECIAL TRENDS

Inpatient Services

Hospitals will continue to provide inpatient services, particularly for specialized treatment and exacerbated secondary and tertiary situations.

Womens Health

Epidemiological studies contribute to knowledge of demographics, environmental and behavioral variables that affect institutional arrangements on the basis of gender, age, or disease. For example, discussion of women's social-health needs now is separated from "medical human" (male) discussions of trends and data. Women's illnesses are being studied, their biological factors viewed in terms of morbidity and mortality. Women's roles in the work-place and as family supporter and caregiver are seen in the context of social-health status. Medical institutions have broadened programs to include, for example, women's health centers that are gender-focused in social-health diagnoses, treatment, and family and work-related problems.

Genetics

The impact of genetics is of major scientific interest. Gene studies are growing exponentially. They are expected to change the course of diagnosis and treatment. However, there is a price to pay. The ethical complications in learning the genetic relationship to probability (risk) of diseases force physicians and their patients to face serious questions about what should be done when the future may be uncertain. Genetics has already begun to cause widespread public and societal concerns.

Geriatric Needs

The elderly are seen within the framework of geriatric team services. Wide diversity exists among the elderly, and the differences need to be understood so service can be designed appropriately. The numbers of elderly are growing and as a group they make the greatest demand on services of any group. More frequently than not, their needs are social and medical which supports the validity of a multiprofessional geriatric team.

Handicapped Issues

The physically handicapped are now being seen in multidisciplinary rehabilitation services. The growth of sports medicine enterprises emphasizes not only maintaining fitness but also repairing damage. New technology and rehabilitative devices, coupled with motivational counseling, are designed to help the handicapped achieve the maximum possible quality-of-life. New behavioral modification techniques support the developmentally disabled, and a growing number of medications deal with mood and behavioral difficulties.

Holistic Care

Medical programs no longer are seen as disease- or disorder-focused but rather as in wellness or holistic services. Care is comprehensive, coordinated, and continuous. This three-dimensional frame of reference supports the notion that care starts at entry to the social-health system and continues into long term care including respite and hospice services as necessary. The three-dimensional framework is fostered by various reform movements occurring in the United States among consumers, women, minorities, the handicapped, and special elderly groups.

THE HEALTH CARE INSTITUTION

Redesigned Structures

The fiscal crisis, reimbursement patterns, new technology, the shift to ambulatory care, and reduction in bed capacity are responsible for a sea change in medical institutions. These institutions are reengineering their systems of services by downsizing and redesigning organizational structures. Hospitals have introduced decentralized units of service (usually related to organ system, disease, or age) that are self-governing. Patient-centered care units appear to be task- and time-oriented. Cost reduction is the stated primary objective as institutions group patients with similar clinical and/or ancillary care needs, bring services closer to the patient, decrease the number of staff involved with patients, and balance staff workload.

The patient-centered units have resulted in the dissolution of central departments in a number of institutions; layoffs of professionals, middle managers, and supervisors; and a shift from professional to in-house trained support personnel who are expected to assume cross-functional duties. The trend affects not only social work departments but a host of nonmedical services, including nursing, pharmacy, laboratory, and other professional services.

Loss of Professionalism

If the patient care unit concept does not safeguard professional assessment and comprehensive inpatient care, the danger exists that the allied health professions will lose professionalism. Professional groups are struggling to secure their services and sustain centralized functions that safeguard quality, secure standards and accountability, and retain selective employment patterns and ongoing professional education. Professionals are educated to serve in the public good and are individual/family-oriented rather than task- and product-focused. Professionals do not merely serve; they define the wants and needs of patients as they serve (Kerson, 1981; p. 229).

Complex of Services

To survive these shifts in service delivery, hospitals must be responsive. Shifting patterns of health care require heightened awareness of trends. Thus hospitals are undertaking new programs that are comprehensive and multidisciplinary in scope and that integrate networks of medical and social services into a social-health system. The health setting will no longer be limited to inpatient programs, but will become a complex entity with an array of facilities and services, including the medical center, nursing homes, public social services, community, family and child support programs, linkage to employer/employee health arrangements, community-based primary care clinics, and managed care enterprises, and prevention, fitness, and wellness programs.

The not-for-profit voluntary medical institution will become a mix of profit and nonprofit enterprises dictated by the payment services of the various reimbursing agents. In addition to creating a self-insured structure with other institutions available to the patients of their attending physicians, they will want to insure their employees for direct health needs as well as create an employee assistance program.

GOVERNMENT ROLES

The future role of government in health care is uncertain. The current trend appears to be toward less involvement of the federal government and increased authority and responsibility of state and local governments. However, states have reacted to their own fiscal crises by imposing restrictions on medical services for the poor, limiting service entitlements, and capping payment for hospital utilization. These limits appear to impose a form of rationing for the poor. Insurance companies and employer-employee benefit programs have limited benefits to include copayments and managed care controls over services.

In the immediate future the government will incur incremental changes only because Congress appears unable to assume responsibility for a national social-health policy. Moreover, many states have shifted from a regulated payment system to deregulation and market negotiations, which most likely will lead to discounted payment arrangements that might compromise service delivery. Financial constraints in local governments will further limit health care for the indigent.

As managed care becomes firmly entrenched in the U.S. health care system, almost half of all insured citizens are in managed care plans (*Hospitals*, Jan 5, 1996; p. 14), which have posed problems involving patient rights, denial of services, doctor gag rules, and too-soon discharges. A public and provider outcry has brought legislative review. New federal policies for Medicare and Medicaid recipients have recently provided protection from denial of care. States are moving to broaden these gains to all insured care recipients.

THE CONSUMER'S VOICE

The voice of the consumer will grow louder and be heard in a variety of movements. Consumer participation in care is a growing phenomenon, as more people take responsibility for their health behavior and focus on prevention to avoid environmental, behavioral, and occupational disorders. Except in very limited ways, medicine is not yet geared to prevention and health education, nor is health promotion a reimbursable service. If consumers are to influence regional services, they must understand health care service and be able to comment on and influence change. An informed public creates informed users who are better able to play an active role in their own care and in changing societal patterns.

Access to health care will continue to be one of the most critical social-health issues and a primary focus of consumer movements. As government, industry, hospitals, and other providers continue to impose barriers to care, consumers must understand monitoring of quality care and standards setting. Public concern has influenced health reform to some degree, as evidenced by recent votes in some state legislatures to safeguard consumer and provider protection in managed care plans.

Rationing of care is a growing public concern. Millions are uninsured and/or underinsured and thus denied care. Public opinion polls demonstrate preference for a universal health coverage that includes basic and essential care; that is, diagnostic, therapeutic, and rehabilitative. The polls also reflect the public's increasing discomfort with taxpayer support of heart transplants for a few, while children and mothers are denied access to care. The public must decide what it wants and what it is willing to pay. A critical need exists to consider a national policy in both social and health terms (Rehr & Rosenberg, 1991; pp. 117–118).

Poverty is the major social problem that must be addressed. The poor are sicker and do not have access to the same level of care as the affluent. Because social welfare, educational opportunities, and health care are intertwined, they should be addressed together. A sound social welfare policy and support of educational opportunities for children are critical to the nation's health. A social welfare policy is essential to lift families out of poverty, assure decent shelter and nutrition, and create job training and work opportunities. Educating consumers can ensure informed decision making about health maintenance and self-care.

Education for health starts in the schoolroom. Educated youths are America's future healthy citizens, informed consumers, and work-oriented individuals and they may be tomorrow's medical care personnel.

Social Work in the New Health Care System

Social workers have achieved important gains in health care, one of which is the ascendancy of its leaders to administrative levels in medical institutions. These leaders bring a social-health and people focus to service. They have applied their professional values to socializing the institution, individualizing care, drawing on family support, and seeking necessary changes in the environment to support new needs while strengthening health care delivery. To be successful in the new health care system, social work leaders and their collegial staff will need to rely on their solid foundation in practice and continue to apply these values.

Leadership matters, and good leaders will be critical to the future of social work in the new health care system. Roles and functions will need to be rethought. A new pattern for social work will need to be set. Social work leaders will deliberate with other professionals as institutions plan expansion beyond their walls to broader roles and functions in the ambulatory arena and in community-based services.

Institutions are expanding their ambulatory linkages to include linkages with primary care, home care programs, respite and hospice care, life-care residencies, and nursing homes. They are affiliating with a range of community-based social agencies as well as community hospitals. Because integrated ambulatory care is seen as cost-effective, financial support for services will come from a host of payers. The new primary care focus will be structured for triage, for acute care, and for the continuum of care. It will provide access to medical care by designated physicians who will follow a patient over time, offering preventive care and selective services that could include referral to medical specialists and other health providers when needed.

New Models of Social Work Service

Social work already has begun to move away from its primary, traditional role of working with hospitalized patients and families and planning their discharge and aftercare. As financing of medical services shifts to outpatient arenas, evidence of support of social work services is occurring: insurers, government, and individuals recognize social work's value and cost-effectiveness. However, new financial arrangements demand that social work develop new organizational and service delivery patterns. Reimbursement revenues are finite; capitation and managed care benefits will fix the dollars available for care.

Social work will be expected to provide viable services within specific, often brief timeframes. Assessment will lead to an agreed-upon plan of service—a contract with the client for the problem to be addressed and for shared responsibilities within a projected visit and/or timeframe. Because of the shortening of length of hospital stay, the shift to ambulatory pre-/posthospital care, and the introduction of a range of one-day ambulatory surgeries and technological treatments, social work will be expected to develop new organizational arrangements that address the social, psychological, and medical problems presented by diverse populations in diverse locations. Preadmission and fast-track triaging will be used to identify individuals with potential aftercare risk. Contractual arrangements with managed care organizations will set prescribed service allocations.

Social work leaders are already introducing models of mixed social work service that include: a combined salaried and private social service for private pay and insured patients; coverage for clientele of group practice physicians for direct referral of their patients; and marketing social work services to affiliated health care providers. We anticipate that social workers will be assigned to selected medical arenas (e.g., patient-centered care units) to be available to clusters of patients with special needs, such as severely ill children in pediatric care and their parents. When recommended, counseling services can be supported under contractual managed care arrangements.

Integrated Services

Social workers will serve as case managers, facilitating selective use of services and resource allocation. As such, they will review service determinants to learn whether client-provider contracts with Medicaid and other insurers are being implemented or require change. Such individual and collective case reviews should lead to new knowledge and to development of new treatment models.

Social workers will become community-based clinicians with one foot in and one foot outside the institution as they provide direct services and serve as consultants and providers regarding the social-health needs of clients within the community network. The institution's services will extend beyond its walls to links with other service systems in the community. Collaboration will lead to networking among social and health agencies. When case circumstances are multifaceted, services will be drawn from many sources. The health care system may support "bundling" of community and health services, coordinated by the hospital.

Consortiums with "packaged care" already are in the marketplace. And social workers already have demonstrated the benefit of their services to patients in group practices and have made inroads in new managed care programs. Because of the breadth and scope of its practice—from services for the geriatric population to women's health to rehabilitation—social work will contribute to the design, the organization, and the implementation of integrated services.

Cost-effectiveness of Service

Social workers will need to look at how they can prevent people from receiving unnecessary and costly medical services. The worried well, the stabilized sick, and those with social ailments will be redirected from medical care to the less expensive social services. Social workers can demonstrate that their services enhance physician productivity and efficiency. They will have a responsibility to define vulnerable populations. High social-risk screening will be expected. Preventive services and those that thwart unnecessary hospitalizations can be offered. As they introduce health promotion and education as well as counseling, social workers will demonstrate the cost-effectiveness of social work services while developing a more educated group of patients for health maintenance and for the utilization of health care.

Shift in Focus

Social work will shift from a diagnosis/disease-illness focus to a focus on individual functional capacities, both physical and social. Social workers will concentrate on social-risk factors as they affect health status. This will require specialized knowledge of the etiology, treatment, and consequences of disease and disability. Major focus will be on risk indicators that relate to chronic illnesses in the elderly, the physically and developmentally handicapped, children who are acutely and chronically ill, and individuals who are terminally ill.

The family and/or an informal network are critical components that affect how the individual copes with illness. Because resources for social work are diminishing in the formal service community, much care will be family-focused strengthening of functioning levels, and will draw largely on clients' informal support systems. Social workers are trained as family-focused therapists. They will be involved with inpatients, but in a limited fashion. Contributions to inpatients and families will be through social diagnosis and motivation, discharge planning, support of home care, rehabilitation, and linkage with essential community-based facilities.

A Case Management Framework

Social work will find a role in case managed care programs, and in those that it will have designed, such as adolescent health services, rehabilitation, employee assistance programs, wellness and prevention programs, and so forth. For those clients who require limited intervention, social work will continue in a range of brief services that are largely concrete and environmental. Inpatient discharge-planning services will be time-limited and brief for those who have positive family and environmental support systems. For those at high social risk, and who need long-term care, triaging and screening will facilitate casefinding.

For certain targeted groups, a continuum of care will need to be prescribed, based on assessment and need. Service determination would fall within a case managed care framework. If care is comprehensive, it would include services such as information and referral, mental health counseling, support services, environmental assistance, and home care. These functions should be negotiated as a covered service. Social workers' knowledge of community social agencies and their ability to network with other facilities will be a requisite in managed care programs so as to service needs, such as via hotlines for crisis intervention. Services may be packaged or bundled with defined reimbursement rates.

Care most likely will be prescribed, limited in service, and limited in the number of contacts. Providers will set critical pathways for patient care. Standardized patterns of care and guidelines will be set by protocols. Like medicine, social work will need to set guidelines for service delivery in prescribed situations. It, too, will argue for the art of practice as an essential component in individualizing client care.

Hospitals will serve a more critically ill population as well as persons with social disorders such as substance abuse and person abuse, which are dollar-productive, reimbursable services. These services will be provided in a system of interdependence with administrators, nurse, doctors, and social workers. Because of the biopsychosocial factors inherent in such disorders, leadership of these programs most likely will be nonmedical.

Special Service Programs

To assist in establishing wellness and health maintenance programs, social workers will need to identify vulnerable and at-risk individuals. Employee assistance programs will grow as institutions recognize the need not only to keep their staffs well and productive but also to help them and their families during illness. Such services will be reimbursable. Employee assistance programs will claim a large number of social workers who will be invested in the problems of the workplace: substance abuse, elder care, child care, stress management, bereavement, and so forth. Hospital employers will seek skilled counselors with business acumen and financial management skills. Industry will employ social workers in case management services for employees, such as elder care for employee parents and consultation about services for social-health concerns that affect absenteeism and performance.

When physicians prescribe counseling services that are endorsed by managed care plans, the services will not be open-ended. Clinical focus will be on a "strengths" perspective which tends to shorten the need for service. No payer will cover ongoing, unlimited care. To achieve cost savings, payers will expect goal-focused, time-limited, and capped services. The benefits of services will need to be substantiated or they will not be reimbursed. Chart notations will be essential; payers will expect documentation of screening, assessment, goals, plans, services provided, and outcomes. Utilization limits will be established and the professions will have to address how much care is enough and find new care methods. Although government support of scientific studies in medicine will be reduced, studies will continue as will development of new technology to enhance diagnostic ability and introduce new treatments. But to be incorporated in the new health care system, new technologies will need to prove themselves to be more cost-effective and beneficial than current procedures and technologies.

Marketing

Social work will need to invest in marketing its services. It will have to strengthen its identity and recognition among constituents, and its clientele will need to acknowledge its value. Institutional providers, community residents, and organizations that pay for services to insured members will want to see the cost-benefit of social work services. The visibility of social work services and their recognized benefits will facilitate marketing. Marketing in the public relations sense will need to be learned.

Quality Improvement, Client Outcomes, and Satisfaction

Comprehensive CQI programs will be expected. This will require systems to gather relevant data. Social workers will need to conduct applied studies. A major means to assure cost-benefit in client services is in measuring social-health outcomes. Outcomes designed to reveal the effects of care not only on physical functioning but on stress and social functioning and on family and others will need to be demonstrated. Patient and family satisfaction with social and other services, while their responses might be considered subjective, are revealing to both payers and providers. Consumers will be asked what they perceive, what their expectations are, what they believe is happening and did happen, and what their satisfaction with outcome is.

Determining client satisfaction with care, correlated with provider satisfaction, will be customary. Casefinding and high social-risk screening to identify vulnerable populations will be expected. Understanding the outcomes of social work services should lead to new treatment models and enhance productivity, and it will uncover the need for continuing education. Routine evaluation of practice and programs will be expected. Practitioner feedback will be essential to ensure continuous improvement in the quality and cost of service. Through patient/family satisfaction studies and demonstrations of services, social work will affirm its contribution to care and health maintenance. Studies of outcomes will influence care and reimbursement. Payers will tie reimbursement to demonstrated effects of therapies.

Participation in Epidemiological Studies

To address populations at risk, social workers will need to be part of multidisciplinary coalitions with public health professionals and other disciplines. At-risk studies not only benefit disease control in developing countries but also help uncover vulnerable individuals and groups in this country. The studies should be regionally based to identify and have a quick impact on priority social problems in the community. Epidemiological studies can help the institution and social work define programmatic needs, casefind prospective users, and evaluate cost-effectiveness. Epidemiological studies help delineate the group at-risk and the patient at high social-risk. A multidisciplinary coalition of professionals, community residents, and industry partners can elicit findings that influence social-health policy deliberation and link social-health care to new knowledge.

At-Home Services and the New Technology

Computer use will be driven by information needs of social work clinicians and administrators. Information will be used to enhance individual performance and integrate departmental requirements. Data will be used for studies that affect service planning. Telecommunications and telephone counseling will be major clinical interventive tools with clients at home or in institutions. The benefits of these tools have been demonstrated and will need to be covered by insurance.

Specialization

Although the trend toward task-oriented and product-trained teams is developing, the long-term continuum of care will require professional skills. Social disorders such as person abuse and substance abuse will require specialized care. Many victims of chronic illness will require ongoing assistance to achieve quality of life. The field of geriatrics has demonstrated that a multiprofessional team is needed to address the myriad problems the elderly face.

Community-Based, Person/Family-Centered Care

Social work will build on collaborative models of service, achieving team leadership and partnership in a community-based, person/family-centered care system with a shared vision. Staff will be culturally diverse, trained to work with cultural diversity. The focus will be on helping clients achieve quality and optimal living patterns. Social workers will work with colleagues in like-minded organizations—networking, building consensus, and setting priorities for community needs. Priorities will be based on research that informs projects for programmatic change. Accountability to clients, the institution, regulators and payers, and the profession will be predicated on the good of the general public as well as the good of the individual.

Leadership

Social work leaders will need to be strong and committed to integration of social-health care with multiprofessional collaboration. Leaders no longer will be caretakers of social services but collaborative organization builders, seekers of information, and partners with staff and colleagues. They must be able to set priorities and encourage staff to join in new visions. They will need to prove the cost-benefits of services to ensure ongoing support for social work service in an integrated social-health system.

Knowledge

What has been critical knowledge for social work practitioners over time remains critical for sound social work services today and tomorrow. Clinical interventions are vital components of the social work enterprise. They will continue to be the essence of practice but will be refined into new roles and functions. As financial issues escalate, triage and assessment skills will need to be enhanced and interventions refined to serve more clients in shorter timeframes. New models of treatment will develop with experience and study. While they continue to focus on individuals and their families in an environmental model, social workers will need to learn the case manager function.

A study of Fortune 500 corporations (National Center for Study of Social Work Practice and Policy, 1992) found that personnel managers and insurance carriers supported social workers as efficient case managers for mental health services and nurses for medical care. To assume case manager roles for disease- and disability-related services, social workers will need to develop greater medical knowledge. A strengths perspective rather than a problem focus will be essential in work with clients in a shared partnership, predicated on the belief that all people and environments possess strengths that can be marshaled to improve the quality of clients' lives (DeJong & Miller, 1995; p. 729). Because it emphasizes what an individual and/or family members did and learned, a strengths perspective lends itself to outcome-focused practice.

Social workers will need to become more knowledgeable about disease, disability, and mental illness, including their direct and indirect consequences, etiology, diagnosis, treatment and medications, and the social and physical functioning potential of clients over time. As they study their practice and engage in selected casefinding, social workers will find themselves more knowledgeable about risk factors and more invested in disease- or disability-specific groups, the frail elderly, and in new women's and children's programs. They must learn to uncover obstacles to access and quality so they can contribute data to substantiate the value of comprehensive biopsychosocial services.

Collaboration and Multidisciplinary Team

These will remain the sine qua non of social work in health care. The ability to collaborate requires professional self-realization and a stance that can support patient advocacy. Social work will need to define its role in an interdependent relationship with other health care providers, not only in service delivery but in program and policy deliberations. Learning to demonstrate the cost-effectiveness of social work services will be essential. Experience with patient-centered care models will prove that task-focused services do not consider the patient's individual social-health needs. As patients, families, doctors, and nurses raise concerns about task-oriented care, consumers will pressure institutions to reintegrate a comprehensive professional service that ensures socially oriented, consumer-friendly care.

Health Education

Most insured contracts of the future will require health education. Many large corporations support employee wellness and fitness programs. Self-care lay education will be a major function of social workers as practitioners in employee assistance programs, as consultants to self-help groups, and as writers for popular magazines.

Fee-for-Service Social Work

Although direct fee-for-service medical care will decline as group practices show steady growth, social work fee-for-service and services incorporated in capitation plans will continue and grow as medical practitioners seek psychosocial counseling for patients. Managed care and other insurers support mental health counseling, the majority of which is performed by social workers. To this end, social workers will need to learn how to contract for services with clients, to clarify client and provider responsibilities, and to set timeframes and fees for service. Social work services will be in group practices with linkages to medical group practices, including those covered by managed care.

Education of Social Workers

Social workers will require knowledge of the medical institution as a system of service and of change. They must develop self reliance as they work with multiple constituencies. As they encounter the corporate world of health care, social workers will need to know financial mechanisms in rate establishment and in reimbursements to providers and institutions. They will need to learn how to contract for social work services with insurers. As they demonstrate that social work services can be cost-effective, they also can demonstrate that social work services can increase the efficiency and productivity of medical care, particularly when social counseling is used with select, vulnerable populations.

CONCLUSION

Without doubt, the changes in health care are dramatic and pivotal. Market forces are transforming the U.S. health care system. How care is financed will affect what will be provided. Pressures and stress on providers will increase. Managed care is expected to support a cheaper, tighter system of services.

As the health system changes, social work in health care has three possible alternatives: reacting by decrying change and portraying it as diminishing quality; sharing others' plans for change; and/or developing innovative programs in partnership with health care colleagues and the community. Evidence exists that social workers can take any one of these three pathways. However, a creative social work leadership in partnership with a creative social work staff will be the catalyst for innovation. Creative leadership will help support an informed public, particularly consumers of social work service, who will agree to and lobby for quality professional care. Professional social workers, particularly in academia, have always argued for a scientific base for practice. This has been as difficult for social work to achieve as it has been for all the behavioral sciences. The many variables and complexities in human behaviors and attitudes make a single practice theory unachievable.

The professional status of social work in health care is not prescribed nor is it tidy. Like the health care delivery system that is changing, social work must change. If it does not, it will have little reason to exist. Change should mean expanded roles: contributing to institutional status, resources, revenues, and programs while supporting access for prospective clients; eliminating fragmentation and obstacles to service; advocating for integration of care; counseling those in need; creating alliances in the community and with other medical institutions; and meeting social-health needs. Social work must be cost-conscious in the changing environment. While safeguarding access, cost-consciousness will foster changing modalities of diagnosis and treatment. High social-risk screening, skilled assessment, client-therapist contracting, brief and group therapies, assisting self-help groups, and health education, are but a few of the areas that will require collaborative consultation skills.

The writings of social work clinicians reflect on a range of practice issues. Social workers' experiences in clinical settings have served them as they observe client needs and recommend programs. Social workers test the quality of service with the means available to them, in particular when they do applied studies and draw on their findings to enhance clinical knowledge and improve care. Collaboration is the essential ingredient in health settings. The recognition that every health concern has a biopsychosocial component has brought an interdisciplinary view to social-health care, which is attested to by an extensive partnership and by jointly authored publications in nonsocial work journals. Social workers have a curiosity about their practice that consists of live interactions, in which they seek to learn what is happening, why it is happening, and what will improve services. Observations prompt the questions that lead to exploration and ideas.

As social workers "reflect-in-action," they move toward managing their professional self and their relationships with others, and toward a self-directed practice. The complexities of the health care institution and the autonomy of medical practice may well have served as models for social workers to seek their own autonomy and self-directedness. That sense of autonomy, combined with knowledge of the medical organization, has allowed them to advocate successfully on behalf of clients. The complexities of illness and disability have helped them value the tenet of family intercession and the meaning of ethical dilemmas and human values. This knowledge of the environment and community resources has informed individual client counseling and helped the institution recognize the need to share health care planning with local residents.

Competency and skill are governed by knowledge and experience, which are in turn enhanced by professional accountability measures and by quality assurance. Social workers have learned to translate institutional missions and goals into services that benefit patients. Social workers also benefit the institution by providing early intervention and easier access to available resources for patients. Their services have had a value-added marketing effect for the institution and have helped reduce the liability of risk.

Social work in the community has created better perceptions of providers and institutions among local residents. As social workers extend their boundaries beyond hospital walls, they see increased interest in their institutions in home care, nursing homes, long-term care, adult day care, schools, special housing, rehabilitation centers, assisted-living care, and primary care, and in wellness, prevention, and employee assistance programs. Social workers have applied health education in the direct client situation and in addressing the lay public.

With all that has been done to enhance the clinical enterprise, both in performance and in administration, social workers have assumed ongoing responsibility for their own continuing education, for educating tomorrow's social workers, and as key contributors to medical education. So much has been done and yet so much lies ahead. These are critical times. How does social work safeguard its gains, thwart attacks on services, ensure professional survival, and promote programs into the next century? It must "come out of the closet," so to speak. It must be visible, market its services, educate its constituencies, participate in policy deliberation and, above all, demonstrate the benefits of service to individuals, families, and the communities, and to their providers and those who regulate and pay for care.

Beyond its commitment to the profession, social work must join in coalitions with other health care professionals to secure and support values in providing human service. As medical care institutions and providers negotiate with insurers and other payers, commitment to the uninsured and underinsured must enter into the deliberations. As downsizing continues, where will further cuts be made? Safeguarding quality and access must be prevalent in commitment to the public. Social work education must move beyond its academic walls and enter into an academic-practice partnership as well as partnership with other health care professionals (public health, in particular), the public, and the business community, that will help social workers face today's social-health problems and the changing environment as well as the fiscal crisis, the reengineering of health-care delivery, and the realities of social work practice for today and tomorrow.

REFERENCES AND BIBLIOGRAPHY

Abramson JS, Mizrahi T (1996). When social workers and physicians collaborate: Positive and negative interdisciplinary experiences. *Social Work, 41*(3):270–281.

Altho SE, Kingberg S (1992). Books helpful to patients with sexual and marital problems: A bibliography. *Journal of Sex and Marital Therapy, 18*(1):70–79.

Ancona-Berk VA, Chalmers TC (1986). An analysis of the costs of ambulatory and inpatient care. *American Journal of Public Health, 76*(9):1102–1104.

Appelbaum J (1993). *How to Get Happily Published.* New York: Harper Collins (paperback edition).

Axinn J, Levin H (1975). *Social Welfare: A History of the American Response to Need.* New York: Harper and Row, p. 94.

Bergman R (1995). Reengineering health care. *Hospitals and Health Networks*, February 5, 28–36.

Berkman B (1975). *The Agency—A Living Laboratory for Research.* Presentation, Council of Social Work Education, Annual Program Meeting, March 4.

Berkman B (1978). *Knowledge Base and Program Needs for Effective Social Work Practice in Health: A Review of the Literature.* Chicago, IL: American Society of Hospital Social Work Directors: 1–91.

Berkman B, Weissman AL (1983). Applied social work research. In R Miller, H Rehr (Eds.). *Social Work Issues in Health Care.* New Jersey: Prentice-Hall.

Berkman B (1996). The emerging health care world: Implications for social work practice and education. *Social Work, 41*(5):542–551.

Berlin SP (1990). Dichotomous and complex thinking. *Social Service Review, 64*(1): 46–59.

Bernstein JE (1983). *Books to Help Children Cope with Separation and Loss,* 2nd ed. New York: Bowker.

Bixby NB (1995). Crisis or opportunity: A health care social work director's response to change. *Social Work in Health Care, 20*(4):3–20.

Blane D (1995). Editorial: Social determinants of health—socioeconomic status, social class and ethnicity. *American Journal of Public Health, 85*(7):903–904.

Blumenfield S (1993). Message from the Director. *The Social Work Connection.* Newsletter of the Social Work Department of the Mount Sinai Medical Center, 2(5).

Blumenfield S (1995). Reflections on effective leadership: Strains and successes, strategies and styles. *Social Work in Health Care, 20*(4):21–37.

Bosch S, Deuschle KW (1989). Social work: An important component of community medicine at Mount Sinai School of Medicine. *The Mount Sinai Journal of Medicine, 56*(6):459–467.

Bracht NF (1978). *Social Work in Health Care: A Guide to Professional Practice.* New York: The Haworth Press.

Briar S (1980). Toward the integration of practice and research. In D Fanshel (Ed.), *Future of Social Work Research.* Washington, DC: NASW.

Campy JS (1995). *Reengineering Business.* New York: Harper Business.

Cannon IM (1952). *On the Social Frontiers of Medicine.* Boston: Harvard University Press, Chapter 1.

Cannon IM (1913). *Social Work in Hospitals.* New York: Russell Sage Foundation.

Carlton TO, Falck HS, Berkman B (1984) The use of theoretical constructs and research data to establish a base for clinical social work in health settings. *Social Work in Health Care, 10*(2):27–40.

Carlton TO (1989). Stand up and cheer! (Editorial). *Health and Social Work, 14*(4): 227–230.

Chavis DM (1993). A future for community psychology practice. *American Journal of Community Psychology, 21*:171–183.

Christ TG (1996). School and agency collaboration in a cost-conscious health care environment. *Social Work, 24*(1/2):53–72.

Davidson KW (1978). Evolving social work roles in health care: The case of discharge planning. *Social Work in Health Care, 4*(1):43–54.

Davidson KW, Clarke S (Eds.) (1990). *Social Work in Health Care: A Handbook for Practice.* New York: The Haworth Press, Parts I and II.

Davis K (1996). *The Future of Health Care. Presentation of Commonwealth Study of Managed Care.* New York: Academy of Medicine, April 13.

DeJong P, Miller SD (1995). How to interview for client strengths. *Social Work, 40*(6):729–736.

Deutsch A (1946). *The Mentally Ill in The United States.* New York: Columbia University Press.

DHEW (1977) *End-Stage Renal Disease Program Guidelines.* Washington, DC: Health Standards and Quality Bureau, Department of Health, Education and Welfare: 1.

Dimond M (1993). Cross-functional management: Strategies for changing times. *Social Work Administration, 19*(4):1–12.

Doernhofer JD, McNamara K (1997). Interview cited in *The New Social Work Connection.* New York: The Mount Sinai Medical Center, April 1997.

Doherty JP, Streeter NA (1993). Progress and limitations in psychotherapy research. *Journal of Psychotherapy, 2*(2):100–119.

Eddleman J, Warren C (1994). Cancer resource center: A setting for patient empowerment. *Cancer Practice, 2*(5):371–377.

Eisenstein EF, Faust JB (1986). The consumer health information library in the hospital setting. *Medical Reference Services Quarterly, 5*(3):66.

Elbow P (1981). *Writing with Power.* New York: Oxford University Press.

Emerson CP (1919) Medical social services of the future. *Hospital Social Services, 1*(4): November.

Epstein I (1995). Promoting reflective social work education. In P Hess, E Mullen (Eds.). *Practice Research Partnership.* Washington, DC: NASW Press: 83–102.

Fischer J (1978). *Effective Casework Practice.* New York: McGraw-Hill.

Flexner A (1915). "Is Social Work a Profession?" National Conference of Charities and Corrections (Proceedings, 42nd Annual Meeting). Baltimore, MD: May 12–19, 587.

Flexner A (1925). *Medical Education, A Comparative Study.* New York: MacMillan Co.

Ford RC, Randolph WA (1992). Cross-functional structures, a review and integration of matrix organization and project management. *Journal of Management, 18*(2):267–294.

Friedson E (1970). *Professional Dominance: The Social Structure of Medicine*, Chicago: Aldine, 88.

Germain CB (1985). *Advances in Clinical Social Work*. Silver Spring, MD: NASW Press.

Germain C, Gitterman A (1987). Ecological perspective. In *Encyclopedia of Social Work*. Silver Spring, MD: NASW Press, 1:488–499.

Goldwater SS (1919). Who started hospital social service? The time, 1636—The place, Paris—The man, Vincent de Paul. *Hospital Social Service*, 1:235–237.

Gould RA (1993). The use of bibliotherapy in the treatment of panic: A preliminary investigation. *Behavior Therapy*, 24(4):241–252.

Gowdy E (1994). From technical rationality to participating consciousness. *Social Work*, 39(4):362–370.

Green RG, Bentley KJ (1994). The attributes, experiences and career productivity of successful social work scholars. *Social Work*, 39(4):405–412.

Greenberg LS, Pinsof WM (1986). Process research: Current trends and perspectives. In LS Greenberg, WM Pinsof (Eds.). *The Psychotherapeutic Process: A Research Handbook*. New York: Guilford Press, 3–19.

Halliday G (1991). Psychological self-help books—how dangerous are they? *Psychotherapy*, 28(4):677–678.

Harbert A, Ginsberg L (Eds.). (1979). *Human Services for Older Adults: Concepts and Skills*. Belmont, CA: Wadsworth.

Harkavy I, Puckett JL (1994). Lessons from Hull House for the contemporary urban university. *Social Service Review*, 9:299–321.

Hirsch J, Doherty B (1952). *The First Hundred Years of The Mount Sinai Hospital of New York, 1852–1952*. New York: Random House: 14–15, 65–75.

Hospitals (1995). Currents, June 20, 12.

Hospitals and Health Networks (1996). January 5: 21–24.

James CS (1985). Ecological approach to defining discharge planning in social work (unpublished paper). School of Social Work, University of Melbourne, Australia.

Jenkins S (1990). The center concept. *Practice and Research Newsletter*, CUSSW-JBFCS, Winter.

Kahn AJ (1969). *Theory and Practice of Social Planning*. New York: Russell Sage.

Katz G, Watt JA (1992). Bibliotherapy: The use of books in psychiatric treatment. *Canadian Journal of Psychiatry*, 37(3):173–178.

Kerson TS (1981). Quotes Everett Hughes on attaining professional status. In *Medical Social Work: The pre-professional paradox*. New York: Irvington Publishers: 151–229.

Kerson T (1981). *Medical Social Work: The Pre-Professional Paradox*. New York: Irvington Publishers.

Kilborne ED (1986). The emergence of the physician-seekers. *Daedalus*, 14(2):43–54.

Kubler-Ross E (1969). *On Death and Dying*. New York: MacMillan.

Kotelchuck R (1992). New York City Health System: A Paradigm under Seige. Presentation, Doris Siegel Memorial Colloquuim. New York: The Mount Sinai Medical Center, April 2.

Lamb HR (1980). Therapist case managers: More than brokers of services. *Hospital and Community Psychiatry*, 31:11.

Lawlor EF, Raube K (1995). Social interventions and outcomes in medical outcomes research. *Social Service Review*, September, 383–404.

Leiby J (1978). *A History of Social Welfare and Social Work in The United States*. New York: Columbia University Press, 74.

Lyons AS, Petrucelli RJ (1978). *Medicine: An Illustrated History*. New York: Harry N. Abrams Inc., 547.

MacEachern MT (1940). *Hospital Organization Management*. Chicago: Physician Record Co., 109–112.

MacKenzie R (1919). Medical social service and the hospital organization. *Hospital Social Service*, 1(2):95.

Mayer JB (1995). The effective health care social work director: Managing the social work department at Beth Israel Hospital. *Social Work in Health Care*, 20(4):61–72.

McDermott W (1969). Keynote Presentation on the Investiture of Dr. Kurt W. Deuschle as the First Lavanburg Professor of Community Medicine, February 14.

McKee S (1989). Bibliotherapy: Looking for Mr. Goodbook. *American Health*, 8(10):42.

Melum MM (1989). Hospitals must change, control is the issue. *Hospitals*, March 1:67–72.

Mickelson JS (1995). Advocacy. *Encyclopedia of Social Work*. Silver Spring, MD: NASW Press, 95–100.

Miller RS, Rehr H (1983). *Social Work Issues in Health Care*. New Jersey: Prentice-Hall: 258.

Nacman M (1977). Social work in health settings: An historical review. *Social Work in Health Care*, 2(4):407–418.

National Center for the Study of Social Work Practice and Policy (1992). Report of the Washington Business Group on Health Study of Social Workers and the Case Management of Catastrophic Care.

O'Leary DS (1991). Accreditation in the quality improvement mold—a vision for tomorrow. *Quality Review Bulletin*, March:72–77.

O'Leary DS (1995). Performance measures: How are they developed, validated, and used? *Medical Care*, 33(1):JS 13–17.

Orlinsky DE, Howard KI (1986). Process and outcome in psychotherapy. In S Garfield, A Bergin (Eds.), *Handbook of Psychotherapy and Behavior Change*, 3rd Edition. New York: Wiley, 311–381.

Pappas G, Queen S, Haden W, Hadden MA, Fischer G (1993). The increasing disparity between socioeconomic groups in the United States, 1960–1986. *New England Journal of Medicine*, 329:103–109.

Pardeck JT, Pardeck JA (1987). Using bibliotherapy to help children cope with the changing family. *Social Work in Education*, 9:107–116.

Pardeck JT (1992). Bibliotherapy and cancer patients. *Family Therapy*, 19(3):223–232.

Pardeck JT (1991). Bibliotherapy and clinical social work. *Journal of Independent Social Work*, 5(2):53–63.

Pearl A, Reissman F (1965). *New Careers for the Poor: The Non-Professional in Human Services*. New York: Free Press, 187–207.

Quackenbush RL (1991). The prescription of self-help books by psychologists: A bibliography of selected bibliotherapy resources. *Psychotherapy*, 28(40):681–687.

Rapaport L (1967). Crisis-oriented short-term casework. *Social Service Review*, 41(March):31–43.

Rehr H (1979). Looking to the Future. In H Rehr (Ed.). *Professional Accountability for Social Work Practice: A Search for Concepts and Guidelines*. New York: Prodist, 150.

Rehr H (1982). *Milestones in Social Work and Medicine*. New York: Prodist: 51.

Rehr H (1985). Medical care organization and the social service connection. *Health and Social Work, 10*(4), 245–257.

Rehr H (1992). Practice use of accountability systems in health care settings and administrative perspective. In AS Grasso, V Epstein (Eds). *Research Utilization in the Social Services: Innovations for Practice and Administration*. New York: Haworth Press, 241–260.

Rehr H, Rosenberg G (1977). Today's education for today's health care social work practice. *Clinical Social Work Journal, 5*(4):242–248.

Rehr H, Rosenberg G (1986). Access to social-health care: Implications for Social Work. In H Rehr (Ed.). *Access to Social Health Care*. Lexington, MA: Ginn Press: 80.

Rehr H, Rosenberg G (1991). Social health care: Problems and predictions. In H Rehr, G Rosenberg (Eds.). *The Changing Context of Social-Health Care*. New York: The Haworth Press.

Research utilization and application of finding. *Research on Social Work Practice,* 2(3), 1992; 363.

Richmond M (1917). *Social Diagnosis*. New York: Russell Sage Foundation.

Rosenberg C (1967). The practice of medicine in New York a century ago. *Bulletin of The History of Medicine,* 41:223–224.

Rosenberg G (1983). Practice roles and functions of the health social worker. In R Miller, H Rehr (Eds.). *Social Work Issues in Health Care*. New Jersey: Prentice-Hall.

Rosenberg G (1987). The social worker as manager in health care settings: An experiential view. In G Rosenberg, SS Clarke (Eds.). Social work in health care management: The move to leadership, social work in health care, 12(3):71–82

Rosenberg G (1994). Social work, the family and the community. *Social Work in Health Care, 20*(1):7–20.

Rosenberg G, Clarke SS (1989). "Findings and Implications." In G Rosenberg, SS Clarke (Eds.). Social work in health care management: The move to leadership. *Social Work in Health Care, 12*(3):143–156.

Rosenberg G, Weissman A (1995). Preliminary thoughts on retaining central social work departments. *Social Work in Health Care, 20*(4):111–116.

Rosner DK (1978). *A once charitable enterprise*. Doctoral dissertation. Submitted at Harvard University, Cambridge, MA, May (mimeo).

Rossen S (1985). *The Role of the Social Worker in Planning*. Chicago: American Hospital Association.

Schon, DA (1983). *The Reflective Practitioner: How Professionals Think in Action*. New York: Basic Books.

Scoggin F, Jamison C, Gochneaur K (1989). Comparative efficacy of cognitive and behavioral bibliotherapy for mildly and moderately depressed older adults. *Journal of Consulting and Clinical Psychology, 57*(23):403–407.

Scoggin F, Jamison C, Davis N (1990). Two-year follow up of bibliotherapy for depression in older adults. *Journal of Consulting and Clinical Psychology, 58*(5): 665–667.

Simmons J (1994). Community-based care: The new health social work paradigm. *Social Work in Health Care, 20*(1):35–56.

Simon EP, Showers N, Blumenfield S, Holden G, Wu X (1995). Delivery of home care services after discharge: What really happens. *Health and Social Work, 20*(1): 5–14.

Smith D, Burkhalter JK (1987). The use of bibliotherapy in clinical practice. *Journal of Mental Health Counseling, 9*:184–190.

Spitzer WJ (1995). Effective leadership: The health care social work director. *Social Work in Health Care, 20*(4):89–109.

Society for Social Work Administrators in Health Care (SSWAHC) (1993). A Special Report of the Health Care Reform Task. Chicago: American Hospital Association.

Starker S (1986). Promises and prescriptions: Self-help books in mental health and medicine. *American Journal of Health Promotion, 1*:19–24, 68.

Starker S (1988). Do it yourself therapy: The prescription of self-help books by psychologists. *Psychotherapy, 25*:142–146.

Stein FT (undated). *The Social Service Department of The Mount Sinai Hospital—A History*, mimeo: 46

Strunk W, White EB. *The Elements of Style*, New York: Macmillan.

Thomas L (1977). On the science and technology of medicine. *Daedalus, 6*(1):42.

Thomlinson R (1984). Something works: Evidence of practice effectiveness. *Social Work*, January-February: 51–56.

USDHHS (1990). Healthy People 2000:National Heart Promotion and Disease Prevention Objectives, DHHS Pub No. (PRS) 912-50212, Washington, DC: Government Printing Office.

USDHHS (1985). Secretary's Task Force on Black and Minority Health: Report. Washington, DC:DHHS.

Verbrugge LM, Patrick DL (1995). Seven chronic conditions and their impact on U.S. adults' activity levels and use of medical services. *American Journal of Public Health, 85*(2):173–182.

Vourlekis BS (1990s). The field's evaluation of proposed clinical indicators for social work services in the acute care hospital. *Health and Social Work, 15*(3):197–206.

Wahl OF (1992). Mental illness topics in popular periodicals. *Community Mental Health Journal, 28*(1):21–28.

Ware JE (1995). What information do consumers want and how will they use it? *Medical Care, 33*(1): JS25-30 Supplement.

Watson AC, Medale EH, Turman LU (1994). How to develop a patient-family resource library. *Cancer Practice, 2*(5):380–383.

Williams LF, Hopps JG (1987). Publication as a practice goal: Enhancing opportunities for social workers. *Social Work, 32*(5):373–376.

Wilson PA (1981). Expanding the role of social workers in coordination of health services. *Health and Social Work, 6*(February):57–64.

Wodarski JS, Feit MD, Green RK (1995). Graduate social work education: A review of 2 decades of empirical research and considerations for the future. *Social Service Review*, March:108–129.

Wood KM (1978). Casework effectiveness: a new look at the research evidence. *Social Work, 23*(6) November:437–458.

Zinsser W (1980). *On Writing Well: An Informal Guide to Writing Nonfiction*. New York: Harper Collins.

Index

('i' indicates an illustration)